# *Quality Assurance*

IN OBSTETRICS AND GYNECOLOGY

## 1989 EDITION

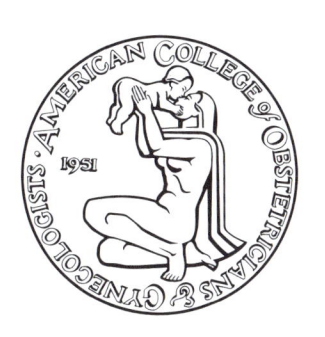

The American College of
Obstetricians and Gynecologists

Members of the American College of Obstetricians and Gynecologists Task Force on Quality Assurance

C. Irving Meeker, MD, FACOG, *Chairman*

W. Baldwin Carey, MD, FACOG
Walter L. Freedman, MD, FACOG
Catherine Heisen, RN, MBA
Douglas R. Knab, MD, FACOG

Joseph D. Millerick, MD, FACOG
William T. Mixson, MD, FACOG
Robert N. Yelverton, MD, FACOG

Staff

John J. Graham, MD, FACOG, *Director, Division of Program Services*
Ann E. Allen, JD, *General Counsel*
John H. Bullock, *Secretary, Quality Assurance*
Pamela S. Cheetham, MPH, *Administrator, Quality Assurance*
Elaine S. Locke, MPA, *Associate Director, Practice Activities*

**Library of Congress Cataloging-in-Publication Data**

Quality assurance in obstetrics and gynecology.
   p. cm.
  Prepared by the American College of Obstetricians and Gynecologists Task Force on Quality Assurance.
  Bibliography: p.
  ISBN 0-915473-10-0
  1. Obstetrics—Quality control.  2. Gynecology—Quality control.
I. American College of Obstetricians and Gynecologists.  Task Force on Quality Assurance.
RG103.4.Q35   1989
362.1'98—dc20                                                           89-31264
                                                                                  CIP

Copyright © May 1989
The American College of Obstetricians and Gynecologists
409 12th Street, SW
Washington, DC 20024-2188

# Contents

|  |  |
|---|---|
| | *Preface*..................................................*vii* |
| chapter 1 | *Overview*................................................*1* |
| | Clinical Indicators ................................. 1 |
| | Criteria Sets........................................... 1 |
| | The System............................................ 2 |
| |    Continuous Monitoring of Department |
| |      Activities (Trends).............................. 2 |
| |    Acquisition of Information from Other |
| |      Hospital Sources.............................. 3 |
| | Conclusion............................................. 4 |
| chapter 2 | *Discussion of Clinical Indicators and* |
| | *Criteria Sets*..........................................*5* |
| | Clinical Indicators ................................. 5 |
| | Criteria Sets........................................... 7 |
| | The Peer Review Process ........................ 8 |
| | Use of Clinical Indicators........................ 9 |
| | Obstetric Clinical Indicators ....................11 |
| | Gynecologic Clinical Indicators ................12 |
| chapter 3 | *Criteria Sets*.........................................*13* |
| | Obstetric Criteria...................................15 |
| |    Antepartum external cephalic version .......15 |
| |    Tocolysis...........................................17 |
| |    Cervical cerclage, prophylactic ...............19 |
| |    Cervical cerclage, therapeutic ................21 |
| |    Cesarean delivery (fetal distress)..............23 |
| |    Cesarean delivery (lack of progress).........25 |
| | Gynecologic Criteria ..............................27 |
| |    Dilation and curettage (abnormal uterine |
| |      bleeding in women of reproductive age)...27 |
| |    Hysterectomy, abdominal or vaginal |
| |      (leiomyomata)...................................29 |
| |    Hysterectomy, abdominal or vaginal |
| |      (chronic pelvic pain) ........................31 |

*iii*

Hysterectomy, abdominal or vaginal
(abnormal uterine bleeding in women of
reproductive age) ............................33
Diagnostic laparoscopy (chronic pelvic
pain) ..............................................35
Cone biopsy of cervix, diagnostic............37
Cone biopsy of cervix, therapeutic ..........39
Surgery for stress urinary incontinence......41
Oophorectomy, unilateral, or ovarian
cystectomy ......................................43

chapter 4 *Administrative Organization of Quality Assurance Activities .............................. 45*
Hospital-wide Quality Assurance Program .......45
Responsibilities of the Medical Staff..........45
Responsibilities of the Hospital
Administration.................................46
Hospital-wide Quality Assurance
Committee.....................................46
Department Quality Assurance Program.........47
Responsibility ...................................47
Implementation and Functioning ............48
Narrative Examples Illustrating Possible Sources
of Quality Assurance Data .......................55

chapter 5 *Corrective Action ................................... 63*
Modifying Clinical Activity of an Individual .....63
Discussion .......................................63
Observation .....................................65
External Peer Review..........................65
Remedial Education...........................66
Proctoring .......................................66
Probation .......................................67
Limiting Privileges.............................67
Revoking Privileges ...........................67
Summary Suspension.........................68
Modifying Clinical Activity of a Department ....68
Due Process.........................................69
Health Care Quality Improvement Act of
1986 ..............................................69
Corrective Action Processes.......................71

chapter 6 *Risk Management Through Quality Assurance............................................. 73*
Quality Assurance and Risk Management ........73
Integration of Quality Assurance and Risk
Management.........................................74
Quality of Medical Records........................75
Qualifications of Medical Staff ....................75
Privilege Delineation ..............................76

*Appendices*  A. The Joint Commission's Agenda for Change .....79
B. Sample Data Collection Forms ....................81
   1. Data Collection Form: Obstetric Indicators................................83
   2. Data Collection Form: Gynecologic Indicators................................85
   3. Department Obstetric Data Summary ..87
   4. Department Gynecologic Data Summary ................................89
   5. Practitioner-Specific Obstetric Statistics ..................................91
   6. Practitioner-Specific Gynecologic Statistics ..................................93
   7. Perinatal Morbidity and Mortality.......95
   8. Quality Assurance Committee Activity Sheet: Individual Case Review .........97
   9. Practitioner Performance Profile (Examples of Important Components)...........................99
   10. Frequency and Sources of Qualitative Data................................. 101
C. Uterine Size and Weight ........................ 103
D. Health Care Quality Improvement Act of 1986 ................................ 105
E. Quality Assurance in ACOG ..................... 117
F. Bibliography......................................... 119
G. Other ACOG Publications....................... 121

*Glossary of Terms* .................................................... **123**

# Preface

The medical specialty of obstetrics and gynecology has a long history of self-analysis. Formal critical examination of obstetric clinical outcomes can be traced back to the inception of maternal mortality committees in the 1920s. Ours was one of the first specialty societies to describe a process of self-assessment for use by its members.

Over the course of more than 15 years, the American College of Obstetricians and Gynecologists (ACOG) has published a number of manuals to inform and assist Fellows who participate in peer review. ACOG publications on this topic have included the following:

- *Indices for Use in the Peer Review of Obstetric/Gynecologic Practice* (1972)
- *Model Screening Criteria for Hospital Admissions in Obstetrics and Gynecology* (1975)
- *Indices for Outcome Audit* (1977)
- *Quality Assurance in Obstetrics and Gynecology* (1981)

The following are other ACOG publications that establish guidelines for this specialty:

- *Standards for Obstetric-Gynecologic Services* (1989)
- *Guidelines for Perinatal Care* (developed with the American Academy of Pediatrics; 1988)

Because quality assurance terminology and review methodology change with some frequency (as does clinical medicine), the issue of peer review must routinely be revisited. For this reason, ACOG formed the Task Force on Quality Assurance. One of the first and primary charges to this group, which began meeting in September 1986, was to determine what issues should be addressed in an ACOG quality assurance publication.

The task force developed the screening clinical indicators and criteria sets in this book by obtaining a consensus among a number of obstetrician-gynecologists on specific clinical issues. Inevitably, neither the discussion of pertinent issues nor the clinical criteria in this document are all-inclusive. Many important procedures and diagnoses have not been included in the criteria sets—in some cases because the technology is quite new and is still evolving rapidly. In other cases, professional judgment regarding efficacy of treatment is too diverse to encapsulate in a brief outline.

The task force has chosen to present an overview of current and widely accepted opinions on ways in which obstetrician-gynecologists who work within a hospital setting can effectively perform ongoing assessment of obstetric and gynecologic clinical care. The narrative sections and the techniques described for assessing clinical care processes and patient outcomes reflect ACOG positions and opinions. Internal review by pertinent ACOG committees has been useful in ensuring that this publication is consistent with other College advisories. Thus, this document is a continuation of the College's effort to facilitate ongoing self-assessment by the practitioners of obstetric and gynecologic medicine.

This manual should be used, just as its predecessors were used, as a guide for health care professionals who are developing specific quality assurance procedures, clinical indicators, and criteria sets to meet their local needs and resources. Economic and geographic factors can influence the availability of resources and may affect both administrative and clinical decision-making; however, it is not only possible but essential that peer review mechanisms and locally developed and agreed-upon clinical standards be used as a means of assessing patient outcomes in every medical setting. This publication is presented to help meet that goal.

# chapter 1
# Overview

*Quality Assurance in Obstetrics and Gynecology* provides a framework around which a practical and useful system can be built to evaluate the obstetric and gynecologic care offered by health care providers. It also suggests methods for the improvement of women's health care. It is intended for all those concerned with maintaining and improving the quality of care received by obstetric and gynecologic patients. This includes not only the physicians who provide and monitor obstetric and gynecologic care in a variety of settings, but also the health care administrators, third-party payers, and all health care professionals who participate in or affect the care of obstetric or gynecologic patients. Most important, this manual is for the women who may not read it but who ultimately will benefit from it.

## CLINICAL INDICATORS

The system suggested in this manual includes a method of monitoring that focuses on a number of activities and outcomes of obstetric and gynecologic care. These events (clinical indicators) can be measured and are used to identify areas that need to be evaluated. The clinical indicators were selected because they are medically important, they occur with sufficient frequency to permit a meaningful review at the practitioner or department level, and they allow some degree of discretion by the health care providers. They are designed to be specific enough for pertinent comparisons on a regional or national basis. The selected indicators should be monitored continuously so that cumulative data will reveal significant trends in practice patterns for individual practitioners and for the department.

The clinical indicators do not measure quality. Rather, they are tools to help identify areas or individual records that should, after initial screening by a nonphysician, be reviewed by quality assurance physicians to determine whether there are problems in the quality of care.

## CRITERIA SETS

The quality of care rendered in any specific situation can be judged only in relation to some acceptable standard of care. Therefore, criteria sets have been developed to define those standards, at least for some of the more common and important diagnoses and procedures of obstetrics and gynecology, so that physicians, health care administrators, and others can refer to them.

It is not the purpose of these standards to establish an optimal level of care. Rather, it is to identify a threshold below which most physicians would agree that the care is substandard and above which there may be several levels of acceptable care. There may also be a variety of clinical approaches, all of which are considered acceptable by some significant portion of the profession. It is recognized that appropriate variations in practice will continue to exist. It is the task and challenge of peer review to determine when identified variations are in fact acceptable, ie, when circumstances dictated that different, but not lower quality, care be provided. The mechanism of peer review will also identify instances when variations in standard care were *not* appropriate and constituted a lower level of medical care quality.

Criteria sets have been developed for only a few of the diagnoses, procedures, and outcomes that might have been chosen. Selection was based partially on repeated inquiries from Fellows of the College about the organization's position on particular diagnoses and procedures (eg, hysterectomy for pelvic pain or for abnormal bleeding). Some important diagnoses, such as pelvic inflammatory disease, are not sufficiently precise to allow application of this type of process with facility. It is intended that conditions and practice activities will continue to be reviewed and that additions, modifications, or deletions will be made as experience dictates. Time and feedback from the users will be the basis for judging the usefulness of this manual. To ensure that there is indeed a reasonable consensus for their use, these criteria sets have been reviewed by the appropriate bodies of the American College of Obstetricians and Gynecologists.

## THE SYSTEM

The quality assurance activities of a department of obstetrics and gynecology as envisioned in this manual include a series of separate, but related, processes.

### Continuous Monitoring of Department Activities (Trends)

The first process involves continuous monitoring of department activities by use of clinical indicators. Some of the indicators may be applicable to hospital-wide activities, while others are department-specific or even subspecialty-specific. To make the screening process as efficient and valuable as possible, the clinical indicators relate to high-volume, high-risk, or problem-prone events. The department may elect to monitor some or all of the events listed among the obstetric or gynecologic clinical indicators in chapter 2. The indicators selected should be used to review the care of all patients in the department. The indicators are not intended to identify every potential maloccurrence or issue of quality of care within the department; rather, they are expected to identify, for physician peer review, records that are most likely to raise questions of quality and to bypass those that are less likely to raise such questions. For example, a significant birth injury, such as Erb palsy, should always be reviewed. The administration of antibiotics for treatment of a postpartum infection should also be identified, because a review of the record is necessary to determine whether the infection is an uncomplicated urinary tract infection or is due to some important deviation from the standard of care. Clinical indicators are designed to be used by a nonphysician, such as a nurse or medical records technician (referred to as the initial abstractor), in screening a large volume of charts.

All charts "flagged" by the clinical indicators or identified through some further screening process by a nonphysician are ultimately reviewed by physicians. As part of the "further screening process," some of the records flagged by the clinical indicators may be reviewed against more specific criteria.

For example, all records flagged by the obstetric clinical indicator "Primary cesarean delivery for failure to progress" (Ob 13), may be checked against four other criteria. First, was the cervix dilated more than 3 cm prior to the cesarean delivery? Second, was the patient in active labor, as evidenced by frequent, regular contractions or by measurements obtained with an intrauterine pressure catheter? Third, if there was any question regarding the quality of labor, were the membranes ruptured and was oxytocin used to augment labor? Fourth, was there any evidence that the cervix had not changed and that the presenting part had not descended during a period of at least 2 hours prior to the cesarean delivery?

The initial abstractor may obtain this information from the patient's medical records. If all four standards were met, physician peer review is not required. If, however, any of these basic standards were not met, the record is held for physician peer review. The use of this method keeps the number of records that require physician peer review manageably small. If the physicians who review the record determine that care was inappropriate, the results of the review are recorded and reported to the head of the department. Depending on the severity of the problem, the department head may institute action. Results are then filed in the provider physician's confidential file.

Clinical indicators can be used to show trends (ie, ongoing or repetitive patterns of care) in an individual practice or in a department. For example, one case in which a hysterectomy is performed for small fibroids may not require action at that time, but the occurrence of several marginal cases in that physician's practice would establish a trend. In some instances, "trending" may reveal areas in which care can be improved, even though the care provided in individual cases may not be considered substandard. Trending may also suggest that the outcomes of a particular diagnosis or procedure are not consistent with those expected. It is the prerogative and responsibility of the department and the institution to determine how this information is used and what follow-up is appropriate. Administrative issues, including those associated with privileges, recredentialing, and due process, are addressed in chapter 5.

The clinical indicators can also be used to create physician profiles, so that each physician's practice pattern for each indicator can be compared to department norms. For example, if the department detects an increase in the number of charts flagged for the gynecologic clinical indicator "Surgery, except radical hysterectomy or exenteration, using two or more units of blood" (Gyn 8) and an investigation of the cases indicates that most were hysterectomies done by the same two physicians, a review of the surgical techniques and indications for surgery used by those two physicians is appropriate. Such profiles should form part of the data base used to make decisions on granting or renewing clinical privileges.

When a more intense focus is warranted, the procedure-specific or diagnosis-specific criteria sets in chapter 3 may be helpful. For example, if the department detects an increase in the number of charts flagged for the clinical indicator "Term infant admitted to a neonatal intensive care unit" (Ob 21) and an investigation indicates that several of these infants were depressed at birth, the department head may decide that a review of intrapartum care is needed. The criteria set "Cesarean Delivery for Fetal Distress" may be helpful for such a review.

### Acquisition of Information from Other Hospital Sources

The second quality assurance process involves the acquisition of information from hospital sources that include those outside the obstetrics and gynecology department. These sources should include the nursing department and committees such as those concerned with surgical review (tissue), infection, transfusion, pharmacy, therapeutics, or medical records (see chapter 4). Reports from sources such as these may identify a problem that requires a focused review of an individual physician's practice or evaluation of the department. For example, if the tissue committee identifies an increase in the number of rather small uteri removed for fibroids, all hysterectomies for this indication may be reviewed. The criteria set "Hysterectomy for Leiomyomata," found in chapter 3, is useful in such a review.

## CONCLUSION

The Joint Commission on the Accreditation of Healthcare Organizations (the Joint Commission) will soon require ongoing monitoring through the use of clinical indicators. Chapter 2 includes obstetric clinical indicators developed by the Joint Commission, plus others that may be worthwhile. Because of Joint Commission mandates—but more important, because of the benefits of continuous monitoring—departments of obstetrics and gynecology should institute ongoing reviews that make use of some or all of the clinical indicators listed in chapter 2. The other sources and methods described earlier will be valuable adjuncts in the evaluation of the quality of care within a department.

Department review should be part of a hospital-wide review system (see chapter 4) and can provide valuable data for creating practitioner profiles. The physician recredentialing and privilege delineation processes (see chapter 4), as well as the hospital's risk management system (see chapter 6), should be closely linked to department quality assurance.

# chapter 2
# Discussion of Clinical Indicators and Criteria Sets

## CLINICAL INDICATORS

Generic screening has become an important mechanism for identifying problem areas in the provision of medical care. The obstetric and gynecologic clinical indicators included in this chapter have been designed to identify diagnoses, procedures, or specific outcomes that can be monitored on a continuing basis. They were selected because they reflect a cross-section of the type of care rendered within the specialty. Indicators should be sufficiently defined so that they can be measured and the results compared with regional or national norms in some meaningful way; thus, deviations from the norm can be recognized. It is a specific goal of the Joint Commission on the Accreditation of Healthcare Organizations (the Joint Commission) to make such comparisons, but it is not the intention of the American College of Obstetricians and Gynecologists (ACOG) to establish or maintain any such regional or national data base.

Clinical indicators may be used to monitor variations in either the processes or outcomes of care. For example, the transfusion of red blood cells (Ob 6) in the course of managing an obstetric patient is part of the process of care, while perinatal mortality (Ob 16) is obviously an outcome. The indicators may also be used to identify individual maloccurrences, such as maternal mortality (Ob 1) or birth trauma (Ob 23). These "sentinel" events should be rare, but they are of sufficient importance for each such event to undergo peer review.

The clinical indicators are only the beginning of the process. They are intended to identify areas that need more detailed review. For example, readmission within 14 days suggests that the patient may have gone home with an unresolved problem (eg, a wound infection) that did not become evident until after discharge. However, the patient may have developed a totally new problem. Even if the problem is related to the care initially rendered, it may not indicate any deviation from the standard of care. Thus, a deliberate decision to discharge a patient 24 hours after delivery may represent hospital policy and may be quite reasonable most of the time, and the occasional readmission related to this early-discharge policy does not represent a deviation from appropriate care. A positive response to an indicator shows that something is different, but not necessarily that the difference is a negative one. It is necessary to determine by some other process, such as a chart review, the reason for this difference. Although the deviation may indeed reflect a lesser quality of care, it may also simply reflect a different population of patients or a policy that is reasonable in most cases. Regardless of the cause, screening by means of the clinical indicators has identified an area where the care provided to the patient preceding (and in some cases following) the event should be examined in greater detail.

The following are some of the specific guidelines used in selecting and defining the two lists of clinical indicators in this chapter:

- Many events selected for screening purposes, such as cesarean delivery (Ob 11–13) or the delivery of premature infants (Ob 14 and Ob 15), occur frequently.
- Some of the events have the potential to affect the patient's health significantly and deleteriously, such as injury to an organ during surgery (Ob 5).
- The events should allow for some discretion in management by the medical team; that is, there should be a possibility of prevention or successful clinical intervention. The initiation of antibiotic therapy (Ob 4) and the prevention or management of eclampsia (Ob 8) are examples of this type of event.
- Some events, although uncommon, are sufficiently important to the patient's health to require identification and review whenever they occur. Birth trauma (Ob 23) and an unplanned admission to a special or intensive care unit (Gyn 5) are two examples of such events.

The goal was to select events that cover a broad range of activities. The assumption behind this approach was that, if these activities have been carried out well, similar activities that have not been measured are likely to have been handled appropriately as well. The two sets of clinical indicators in this chapter are not all-inclusive, nor are they the only ones that might have been selected. They were chosen from a variety of sources. Several are generic screening criteria that have been used by individual hospitals and have appeared in the literature for a number of years. Others were developed by a task force that was established by the Joint Commission to identify obstetric clinical indicators for use in the Joint Commission accreditation process. These indicators have been included in the ACOG obstetric clinical indicator list so that users of this screen can gain familiarity with future Joint Commission monitoring procedures. An institution can add or delete clinical indicators as seems appropriate in that setting.

The clinical indicators are intended to address the question of outcome wherever possible. This is consistent with the Joint Commission Agenda for Change (see appendix A for a brief overview). A primary question regarding evaluation is not only whether an institution is capable of delivering quality care, but also whether it actually is delivering quality care. The Joint Commission clinical indicators included here are limited to those in the field of obstetrics and, therefore, are less comprehensive than the ACOG list.

The various sample forms contained in appendix B illustrate formats in which aggregated department-wide data and physician-specific data collected through the use of the clinical indicators, as well as from the department's regular sources of statistical data, can be recorded. These data should include the department's and the individual staff members' total volume and frequency of important procedures and occurrences. In other words, the summary data sheets are tools to examine trends in care. They should be used to compare performance over a period of time; quarterly (or at least annual) analysis of individual and department activity is recommended.

Many of the clinical indicators are, by design, generally more sensitive than specific. This creates a practical problem in linking the use of the clinical indicators to physician chart review. In some situations, the clinical indicators by themselves will flag more charts than are either necessary or desirable for a physician review process. To address this problem, the department may wish to use a trained nonphysician for the initial review of any records that are flagged by the clinical indicator screen. This individual should be trained to recognize the records that are likely to represent quality of care issues and to prepare a list of the records that should be examined by the quality assurance committee. As an alternative, specific exclusionary qualifiers can be introduced. For example, the clinical indicator "In-hospital initiation of antibiotics 24 hours or more following term vaginal delivery" (Ob 4), modified with "except in cases of endometritis in which the patient's temperature returns to normal within 36 hours of treatment" could be used by the abstractor as a second screen for those records that are flagged by the first screen. With this approach, only the more serious infections would be reviewed. Thus, the clinical indicators may be modified to fit the needs of a particular department at both the practical and theoretical level.

## CRITERIA SETS

The second part of this quality assurance system is based on criteria sets. To measure or evaluate any activity, it is necessary to compare it to some acceptable standard. Thus, one important objective of this manual is to provide basic guidelines about what should and should not be done in the diagnosis and management of some obstetric and gynecologic conditions.

These guidelines have been called criteria sets. They differ from the clinical indicators in that the criteria sets are intended to help in the evaluation and measurement of the quality and appropriateness of care, not just in the identification of areas for further study.

With these criteria sets, reviewers should be able to judge whether proper care has been delivered and, if not, why not.

There were two essential considerations in creating the criteria sets. First, the standards had to be generally accepted as appropriate. Therefore, the criteria were constructed to describe a *threshold of provider activity below which most physicians would agree that care was substandard*. It is recognized that above this threshold there may be several levels of acceptable care, as well as different, but equally acceptable, approaches to care.

Second, to ensure insofar as possible that the criteria chosen are appropriate, each set was reviewed by the appropriate ACOG committees and commissions. (The same peer review process was used for the clinical indicators.) In addition, all relevant ACOG publications (eg, Technical Bulletins and the *Guidelines for Perinatal Care*) have been used in the development of the criteria sets. Despite this extensive peer review process, it is expected that the criteria will be revised and expanded through continuing dialogue within the specialty. Updates and additional criteria sets will be disseminated as they are developed.

*Discussion of Clinical Indicators and Criteria Sets*

Some may criticize the criteria sets as being less rigorous than is optimal. This may be a valid concern. If a department desires to increase its requirements in a way that transforms the generally acceptable criteria into something more rigorous, additional requirements should be established locally.

## THE PEER REVIEW PROCESS

Areas of potential concern may be identified in a variety of ways. The use of the clinical indicators included in this chapter is one method of identifying an area for review, but other screening systems may be used as well. Furthermore, any of the standard risk management or quality assurance mechanisms used in most hospitals may also focus attention on areas of care that should be evaluated. These mechanisms include, but are not limited to, the activities of the surgical review committee (tissue and transfusion), infection control committee, and pharmacy committee; incident reports; and observations of the patient care committee.

Once an area of concern has been identified by any means, it is the responsibility of the institution to conduct a more detailed study to determine the nature of the problem and the reasons behind it. This can be accomplished by means of a focused, retrospective review. Designed to assist in this process, the diagnosis-specific and procedure-specific criteria sets list a series of steps or actions that should occur before a diagnosis is made or a procedure is performed. These standards may serve as a basis for an evaluation of records in the focused review process.

Local standards may be added to these criteria sets if desired. For example, the criteria set for hysterectomy for abnormal uterine bleeding calls for endometrial sampling prior to the hysterectomy. Many physicians believe that, because of its possible therapeutic benefit, dilation and curettage (D&C) should be required. The decision to require D&C rather than just an endometrial sample should be made at the local level.

Some activities should not occur in association with a particular diagnosis or procedure. If a cesarean delivery is performed for the indication "lack of progress," for example, the patient should not have been in the latent phase of labor; in this case, lack of adequate labor may have been the problem. The abstractor can determine whether the patient was in the latent phase by noting whether the cervix was dilated at least 3 cm in a nullipara or 4 cm in a multipara prior to the delivery. Likewise, tocolysis for preterm labor is contraindicated if severe hemorrhage, fetal demise, or severe pregnancy-induced hypertension is present. These and similar standards from the criteria sets can form the basis for a focused review.

Each institution should be able, through a review of the patient record, to determine whether the care provided has met the minimum criteria. Either a manual system or a computer program may be used for this record review. More sophisticated data can be generated more easily and more directly if a computer program is used, but this is not essential to make the system work. The clinical indicators selected can be reviewed on the record of every patient discharged from the department of obstetrics and gynecology. The abstractor should indicate the reason for each positive response (eg, birth trauma [Ob 23], Erb palsy). This information can be tracked for each physician for feedback and for trending.

Any records flagged by the clinical indicators should be reviewed by a local quality assurance panel before the care provided is judged to be substandard. This physician panel may use the criteria sets in evaluating care. If the panel concludes that a record reflects care of poor quality, the head of the department and the provider physician should review the record to ensure that the information in the record is complete and accurate. If the record is inaccurate or incomplete, the problem may simply be one of poor documentation rather than substandard care; but this, too, is a problem and should be identified as such. If the care has in fact been substandard, the head of the department will already have begun the process of corrective action and education by reviewing the facts with the provider physician.

The result of this review by the committee and the head of the department should become part of both the department's and the individual's quality assurance files. It is the responsibility of the institution and the department to decide at what point the frequency and seriousness of adverse judgments require specific follow-up action and to determine what such action should be. These issues are discussed in more detail in chapter 5. Education should be the initial response to most deviations from the standard of care, whether the deviation occurs within the activity of the department as a whole or within the practice of an individual physician. The quality assurance committee or the department head may recommend specific topics to be addressed during grand rounds or other educational programs when a problem involves several department staff members. Continuing medical education may be recommended to meet the educational needs of an individual physician.

It is necessary to maintain a record of all actions reviewed in order to identify trends that are collectively important, even though the care provided in individual cases may not have been judged to be substandard or to require corrective action. With all this information, both institutional and individual data bases are developed. These data can then be compared with regional and national thresholds, when available, to determine the quality of care associated with specific diagnoses and procedures in the department.

## USE OF CLINICAL INDICATORS

Forms (similar to those illustrated in appendices B-1 and B-2) should be created to record data on all obstetric and gynecologic indicators selected by the department for monitoring. The medical records department should be asked to place the records for all patients discharged from the obstetric and gynecologic department in a single location each day, as soon after discharge as the basic information is complete. Because of billing requirements, most institutions can do this within 5 days of discharge. With obstetric patients, it is essential that the records for mother and baby be placed together if they are discharged on the same day.

The abstractor assigned to collect the data from patient records should do so every day, or at least every other day, so that the charts will not be removed and have to be relocated later. Equally important, this system of collecting data on a regular basis ensures that the number of records will be manageable and that only a short time will be needed to complete the task; this avoids tedium and ensures a more accurate collection of data. The abstractor should have, at a minimum, familiarity with medical records and medical terminology; ideally, the abstractor also would have significant experience in the specialty of obstetrics and gynecology. Once familiar with the system, the abstractor can collect the needed data from both the maternal and infant records, if they are available together, in less than 5 minutes. When the data for a month have been recorded, usually by the 10th of the following month, the data collection forms are given to the individual responsible for quality assurance activity in the department. In some institutions, the data are placed in a computer, where various programs make further use of the data to generate a variety of reports with a minimum effort on the part of the quality assurance personnel. In a small service (ie, 500 or fewer deliveries per year), these data can easily be counted by hand to obtain the basic reports needed to develop department and individual practitioner profiles. Even in a larger service (eg, 3,000 deliveries), the data can be managed by hand in several hours per month. Samples of formats for department and practitioner-specific data summaries are included in appendices B-3 through B-7.

It is suggested that the clinical indicators be used in two ways. First, the indicators are used to flag the records that should be rechecked by a physician or experienced reviewer to determine whether there is an issue of quality in the care rendered. Those records are then held for the quality assurance committee, which makes the actual judgment on the quality of care. It should be anticipated that only a small percentage of all records will be flagged and that the majority of those will not raise serious questions of quality. The number of records for committee review should be small.

Second, the clinical indicators are used in trending and in developing practitioner performance profiles. It is essential that the abstractor identify the physician directly involved in a patient's care when a particular incident is in question. This is not necessarily the patient's physician, who may not have been on call when the incident in question occurred. Because only five to 10 of the indicators are likely to account for most of the flagged records, physician-specific profiles can be developed rapidly. Even though complications may be difficult to explain in individual cases, recording the code of the physician who actually provided the care in each case makes it possible to determine whether the rate of complications among the patients of a particular physician is consistently higher than that among the patients in the department as a whole.

The impetus for department or individual reviews may come from a variety of sources. An increase in the department's rate of perinatal mortality or in its rate of cesarean deliveries suggests the need for a focused review. If birth trauma occurs more often among a particular physician's patients than among the department's other patients, the records of that physician's patients must be examined immediately. The department must decide whether the occasional removal of a small uterus for fibroids is acceptable or whether it is necessary to defend the removal of each normal uterus before the quality assurance committee or the department head. (Appendix C includes a table of uterine size and weights which may be helpful in discussing this issue.) It is the responsibility of each institution and department to decide what their tolerance thresholds will be.

**OBSTETRIC CLINICAL INDICATORS**

A. Maternal Indicators
  *1. Maternal mortality
  *2. Unplanned readmission within 14 days
   3. Cardiopulmonary arrest
  *4. In-hospital initiation of antibiotics 24 hours or more following term vaginal delivery
   5. Unplanned removal, injury, or repair of organ during operative procedure
  *6. In-hospital maternal red blood cell transfusion or hematocrit of less than 22 vol% or hemoglobin of less than 7.0 g or decrease in hematocrit of 11 vol% or hemoglobin of 3.5 g or more
  *7. Maternal length of stay more than 5 days after vaginal delivery or more than 7 days after cesarean delivery
  *8. Eclampsia
   9. Delivery unattended by the "responsible" physician†
  10. Postpartum return to delivery room or operating room for management
  *11. Induction of labor for an indication other than diabetes, premature rupture of membranes, pregnancy-induced hypertension, postterm gestation, intrauterine growth retardation, cardiac disease, isoimmunization, fetal demise, or chorioamnionitis
      a. Cesarean delivery required
  12. Primary cesarean delivery for fetal distress
  *13. Primary cesarean delivery for failure to progress
  *14. Delivery of an infant with a birth weight less than 2,500 g or respiratory distress syndrome after planned repeat cesarean delivery‡
  *15. Delivery of an infant with a birth weight less than 2,500 g or respiratory distress syndrome following induction of labor‡

B. Neonatal Indicators
  *16. Perinatal mortality of a fetus or infant surviving less than 28 days and weighing 500 g or more at delivery
  *17. Intrapartum death, in hospital, of a fetus or infant weighing 500 g or more
  *18. Neonatal mortality of an inborn infant§ with a birth weight of 750–999 g in an institution with a neonatal intensive care unit (NICU)
  *19. Delivery of an infant weighing less than 1,800 g in an institution without an NICU
  *20. Transfer of a neonate to an NICU in another institution
  *21. Term infant admitted to an NICU
  *22. Apgar score of 4 or less at 5 minutes
  *23. Birth trauma (#767 in ICD-9-CM directory), such as shoulder dystocia, cephalohematoma, Erb palsy, and clavicular fracture but not caput
  *24. Diagnosis of fetal "massive aspiration syndrome #770.1 in ICD-9-CM"
  *25. Inborn term infant with clinically apparent seizures recorded prior to discharge

*Indicator was one of the Joint Commission's clinical indicators for obstetrics that were being field tested in spring 1989 when this manual went to press. These may be modified somewhat in summer 1989 based on findings from field testing.

†To be defined by each institution.

‡The same exception as for Ob 11 might be used to explain reasons for repeat cesarean delivery or elective induction.

§An inborn infant is one born in this hospital rather than transferred from another institution.

## GYNECOLOGIC CLINICAL INDICATORS

1. Unplanned readmission within 14 days
2. Admission after a return visit to the emergency room for the same problem
3. Cardiopulmonary arrest
4. Occurrence of an infection not present on admission
5. Unplanned admission to special (intensive) care unit
6. Unplanned return to operating room for surgery during the same admission
7. Ambulatory surgery patient admitted or retained for complication of surgery or anesthesia
8. Gynecologic surgery, except radical hysterectomy or exenteration, using 2 or more units of blood or postoperative hematocrit of less than 24 vol% or hemoglobin of less than 8 g
9. Unplanned removal, injury, or repair of organ during operative procedure
10. Initiation of antibiotics more than 24 hours after surgery
11. Discrepancy between preoperative diagnosis and postoperative tissue report
12. Removal of uterus weighing less than 280 g for leiomyomata
13. Removal of simple cyst or corpus luteum of ovary
14. Hysterectomy performed on woman younger than 30 except for malignancy
15. Gynecologic death

# chapter 3
# Criteria Sets

The criteria sets in this chapter have been constructed to reflect threshold levels of care; thus, they represent the *minimum* level of care acceptable in the performance of the specific procedures in question. Care should not be less comprehensive.

It is obvious that the care of individual patients will fail to meet these criteria on occasion. Such a failure does not, in itself, always indicate that substandard care has been rendered. It is, however, clearly the responsibility of the provider physician to demonstrate why care for a particular patient is different and should be viewed as an acceptable variation from established criteria.

Individual hospitals are encouraged, if their local resources permit and such care is indicated by patients' conditions, to offer substantially more sophisticated care than that outlined in these criteria. *Care that is more sophisticated or intense than the basic care outlined in the criteria sets may not represent and should not be automatically construed to represent an inappropriate or unnecessary utilization of resources.*

A higher level of care may be necessary in the presence of comorbidity. Other significant physical conditions, such as a chronic illness, are apt to increase the amount, level, and perhaps duration of medical care needed by any individual patient. These criteria have been designed for a hypothetical situation in which a patient is free of all physical and psychologic conditions except that for which each individual criteria set describes care.

Within the criteria sets are found corresponding ICD-9-CM code numbers (for procedures and diagnoses). Because these codes are not always closely correlated with the categories used in this manual, each department of medical records should carefully record which, if any, code numbers are used in selecting charts to be included in reviews. If there is no common agreement on the composition of code categories, use of the codes may result in more confusion than clarity.

**Procedure:** Antepartum external cephalic version (no code)

**Indication:** Breech or transverse lie (652.2 and 652.3)

**Confirmation of Indication:**
1. Pregnancy of 36 weeks or more
2. Ultrasound examination

**Actions Prior to Procedure:**
1. Perform fetal assessment study
2. Ensure availability of hospital staff and facilities for immediate cesarean delivery

**Actions During and/or Following Procedure:**
1. Monitor fetal heart rate
2. Monitor procedure with ultrasound
3. Prior to discharge, observe patient for at least 1 hour for pain, bleeding, or labor

**Contraindications:**
1. Compromised fetus
2. Oligohydramnios
3. Placenta previa
4. Premature rupture of membranes
5. Multiple gestation

Unless otherwise stated, **each** numbered and lettered item (except contraindications) **must** be present.

May 1989

**Procedure:** Tocolysis (99.29)

**Indication:** Preterm labor (644.0)

**Confirmation of Indication:**
1. Gestational age of at least 20 weeks but less than 37 weeks, confirmed by dates or ultrasound examination
2. Regular uterine contractions at frequent intervals, preferably documented by tocodynamometer
3. Documented cervical change or appreciable cervical dilation or effacement

**Actions Prior to Procedure:**
1. Advise bed rest
2. Administer fluids intravenously for hydration
3. Assess gestational age and fetal status
4. Perform urinalysis

**Actions During Procedure:**
1. Monitor fluid intake and urine output
2. Observe patient for development of pulmonary edema

**Contraindications:**
1. Maternal
    a. Chorioamnionitis
    b. Severe antepartum vaginal bleeding
    c. Severe pregnancy-induced hypertension (severe preeclampsia)
    If beta-mimetics are used:
    d. Significant cardiac disease
    e. Pulmonary hypertension
    f. Uncontrolled hyperthyroidism
    g. Uncontrolled diabetes
2. Fetal
    a. Fetal demise
    b. Fetal anomaly incompatible with life
    c. Other fetal conditions in which prolongation of the pregnancy is detrimental to fetal life

Unless otherwise stated, **each** numbered and lettered item (except contraindications) **must** be present.

May 1989

**Procedure:** Cervical cerclage (67.5), prophylactic*

**Indication:** Incompetent cervix (654.53)

**Confirmation of Indication:**
Presence of either number 1 or number 2
1. History of prior pregnancy in which patient had classic signs of incompetent cervix
2. Prepregnancy physical findings suggesting possible cervical incompetence in a patient with history of a prior spontaneous, midtrimester abortion. At least one of the following should be present:
    a. Ability to introduce no. 8 Hegar dilator through internal os when patient is not pregnant
    b. Withdrawal of Foley balloon with 2–3 ml of water through cervical canal with minimal resistance
    c. Hysterosalpingogram demonstrating cervical funneling
    d. Clinical evidence of significant cervical anomalies suggestive of in utero exposure to diethylstilbestrol (DES)
    e. Clinical evidence of extensive obstetric trauma to cervix

**Action Prior to Procedure:**
Confirm fetal age and status by ultrasound examination

**Contraindications:**
1. Chorioamnionitis
2. Premature rupture of membranes
3. Fetal anomaly incompatible with life
4. Fetal demise

---

*Evaluation of the quality of care provided with this procedure, when performed for the indication listed, will be possible through "trending." See the discussion of trending in chapter 1.

Unless otherwise stated, **each** numbered and lettered item (except contraindications) **must** be present.

May 1989

**Procedure:** Cervical cerclage (67.5), therapeutic

**Indication:** Incompetent cervix (654.53)

**Confirmation of Indication:**
1. Premature effacement and/or dilation of cervix in absence of labor prior to 28 weeks of gestation

and/or

2. Sonographic evidence of cervical funneling, especially in a patient with prior history of midtrimester delivery

**Action Prior to Procedure:**
Confirm fetal age and status by ultrasound examination

**Contraindications:**
1. Preterm labor
2. Active uterine bleeding
3. Chorioamnionitis
4. Premature rupture of membranes
5. Fetal anomaly incompatible with life
6. Fetal demise

Unless otherwise stated, **each** numbered and lettered item (except contraindications) **must** be present.

May 1989

**Procedure:** Cesarean delivery (74 all; subcode dependent on which type of procedure is used)*

**Indication:** Fetal distress (656.33 FD affecting management of mother antepartum) (656.31 FD affecting management of mother delivered)†

**Confirmation of Indication:**
Presence of 1 or 2 or 3 or 4
1. Persistent‡ severe, variable decelerations
2. Persistent‡ and nonremediable late decelerations
3. Persistent‡ severe bradycardia
4. Scalp pH less than 7.2

**Actions Prior to Procedure:**
1. Reposition patient
2. Administer oxygen by mask
3. Perform vaginal examination to check for prolapsed cord
4. Perform vaginal examination to rule out imminent‡ vaginal delivery
5. Initiate preoperative routines
6. Monitor fetal heart tones (by continuous electronic monitoring or by auscultation) immediately prior to preparation of abdomen
7. Ensure that qualified personnel‡ are in attendance for resuscitation and care of newborn

---

*Evaluation of the quality of care provided with this procedure, when performed for the indication listed, will be possible through "trending." See the discussion of trending in chapter 1.

†The term "fetal distress" is included here because it is still commonly used. It is not, however, a sufficiently accurate description of fetal condition. The term "abnormalities in fetal monitoring" better reflects the indication for cesarean delivery herein described.

‡Locally acceptable definitions for persistent, imminent, and qualified personnel should be agreed upon by authorities at each institution.

Unless otherwise stated, **each** numbered item **must** be present.

May 1989

**ACOG OBSTETRIC CRITERIA**

**Procedure:** Cesarean delivery (74 all; subcode dependent on which type of procedure is used)*

**Indication:** Lack of progress (failure to progress) (660.61—failed trial of labor; 662.11—long labor)

**Confirmation of Indication:**
1. No change in either dilation of cervix or descent of presenting part after at least 2 hours of active labor
2. Active labor indicated by
    a. Cervix dilated to at least 3 cm in nullipara or 4 cm in multipara
    b. Contractions at least every 2–3 minutes
    c. Strength of contractions at least 50 mm Hg internal pressure as measured by intrauterine catheter or inability to indent fundus on palpation

**Actions Prior to Procedure:**
1. Rupture membranes
2. In absence of active labor, administer oxytocin to augment labor
3. Obtain anesthesia consultation and evaluation
4. Type and screen blood sample
5. Monitor fetal heart tones (by continuous electronic monitoring or by auscultation) immediately prior to preparation of abdomen
6. Ensure that qualified personnel† are in attendance for resuscitation and care of newborn
7. Perform vaginal examination just prior to surgery

---

*Evaluation of the quality of care provided with this procedure, when performed for the indication listed, will be possible through "trending." See the discussion of trending in chapter 1.

†To be determined by each institution.

Unless otherwise stated, **each** numbered and lettered item **must** be present.

May 1989

**Procedure:** Dilation and curettage (D&C 69.09)

**Indication:** Abnormal uterine bleeding in women of reproductive age (626 all, except 626.0, 626.1, 626.5, 626.7)

**Confirmation of Indication:**
History of abnormal uterine bleeding persisting for two cycles or more*

**Actions Prior to Procedure:**
1. Obtain endometrial sample in office†
2. Determine that attempted hormone treatment (estrogen/progestogen) was not successful
3. Consider metabolic disturbances
4. Consider bleeding diathesis
5. Consider pregnancy

**Contraindication:**
Acute pelvic inflammatory disease

---

*Except for profuse bleeding requiring treatment.

†Except when unable to perform sampling in office.

Unless otherwise stated, **each** numbered and lettered item (except contraindication) **must** be present.

May 1989

**Procedure:** Hysterectomy, abdominal (68.4) or vaginal (68.5)

**Indication:** Leiomyomata (218.0–218.9)

**Confirmation of Indication:**
Presence of 1 or 2 or 3 or 4
1. Asymptomatic myomata associated with a uterine size equal to or larger than that after 12 weeks of gestation,* determined by physical examination or ultrasound examination
2. Excessive uterine bleeding evidenced by *either* a or b:
    a. Bleeding for more than 8 days during more than a single cycle and profuse bleeding† requiring additional protection
    b. Anemia due to acute or chronic blood loss
3. Pelvic discomfort caused by myomata associated with a uterine size equal to or larger than that after 12 weeks of gestation
    a. Acute and severe
    b. Chronic lower abdominal or low back pressure
    c. Bladder pressure with urinary frequency not due to urinary tract infection
4. Rapid growth in size of uterus/myomata, to a point equal to or larger than uterine size after 12 weeks of gestation

**Actions Prior to Procedure:**
1. Confirm by cytologic study the absence of cervical malignancy
2. Obtain endometrial sample or perform D&C (when abnormal bleeding is present)
3. Correct anemia
4. Consider patient's medical and psychologic risks concerning hysterectomy

**Contraindication:**
Desire to maintain fertility, in which case myomectomy may be considered

---

*Transverse measurement of at least 8 cm or weight of 280 g or more (see appendix C).

†For example, large clots, gushes, limitations on activity.

Unless otherwise stated, **each** numbered and lettered item (except contraindication) **must** be present.

May 1989

**Procedure:** Hysterectomy, abdominal (68.4) or vaginal (68.5)*

**Indication:** Chronic pelvic pain in the absence of significant pathology (625.9)†

**Confirmation of Indication:**
1. No significant pathology found on laparoscopic examination
2. Presence of pain for more than 6 months with negative effect on patient's quality of life

**Actions Prior to Procedure:**
1. Document failure of a therapeutic trial with, for example, one or more of the following:
   a. Oral contraceptives
   b. Diuretics
   c. Nonsteroidal antiinflammatory drugs
   d. Induced amenorrhea
2. Evaluate the following systems as possible sources of pelvic pain:
   a. Urinary
   b. Gastrointestinal
   c. Musculoskeletal
3. Evaluate patient's psychologic and psychosexual status and counsel
4. Confirm by cytologic study the absence of cervical malignancy

**Contraindication:**
Desire to maintain fertility

---

*Evaluation of the quality of care provided with this procedure, when performed for the indication listed, will be possible through "trending." See the discussion of trending in chapter 1.

†Other diagnoses that should also be evaluated according to these criteria include pelvic congestion (625.5); pelvic varices (456.5); uterine retroversion (621.6); congenital anomalies (752.3); mild endometriosis (617–617.9); minimal pelvic adhesions (614.6); broad ligament window (620.6); first-degree uterine prolapse (618–618.9); and mild adenomyosis (617.0).

Unless otherwise stated, **each** numbered and lettered item (except contraindication) **must** be present.

May 1989

**Procedure:** Hysterectomy, abdominal (68.4) or vaginal (68.5)*

**Indication:** Abnormal uterine bleeding in women of reproductive age (626 all, except 626.0, 626.1, 626.3, 626.5, 626.7)†

**Confirmation of Indication:**
1. History
   a. Excessive uterine bleeding
      1. Bleeding for more than 8 days during more than a single cycle
      2. Profuse bleeding requiring additional protection‡
   b. No history of a bleeding diathesis or use of medications that may cause bleeding
   c. Negative effect on patient's quality of life
2. Failure to find on physical examination uterine or cervical pathology that would cause abnormal bleeding
3. Laboratory data
   a. No finding of endometrial neoplasia
   b. No malignancy found in cytologic studies of cervix
4. No finding of endometrial polyps (by D&C, hysteroscopy, or hysterogram)

**Actions Prior to Procedure:**
1. Consider patient's medical and psychologic risks concerning hysterectomy
2. Determine that attempted hormone treatment (estrogen–progestogen) was not successful

**Contraindication:**
Desire to maintain fertility

---

*Evaluation of the quality of care provided with this procedure, when performed for the indication listed, will be possible through "trending." See the discussion of trending in chapter 1.

†Other diagnoses that should also be evaluated according to these criteria include menorrhagia (626.2, 627.0), hypermenorrhea (626.2), dysfunctional uterine bleeding, menometrorrhagia (626.2), and polymenorrhea (626.2).

‡For example, large clots, gushes, limitations on activity.

Unless otherwise stated, **each** numbered and lettered item (except contraindication) **must** be present.

May 1989

**Procedure:** Diagnostic laparoscopy (54.21)*

**Indication:** Chronic pelvic pain (625.9)

**Confirmation of Indication:**
   Pelvic pain for more than 3 months without demonstrated cause

**Actions Prior to Procedure:**
1. Obtain meticulous history concerning pain
2. Evaluate the following systems as possible sources of pelvic pain:
   a. Gastrointestinal
   b. Lower urinary
   c. Musculoskeletal

**Contraindication:**
   Severe cardiorespiratory disease

*Evaluation of the quality of care provided with this procedure, when performed for the indication listed, will be possible through "trending." See the discussion of trending in chapter 1.

**Unless otherwise stated, each numbered and lettered item (except contraindication) must be present.**

May 1989

**Procedure:** Cone biopsy of cervix, diagnostic (67.2)

**Indication:** Cervical intraepithelial neoplasia (233.1, 622.1)

**Confirmation of Indication:**
Presence of 1 or 2 or 3 or 4 or 5
1. Microinvasive carcinoma of cervix found on colposcopically directed biopsy
2. Cervical intraepithelial neoplasia found on endocervical curettage
3. Cervical cytology report suggesting disease more severe than that found by colposcopically directed biopsy
4. In situ adenocarcinoma of cervix
5. Inability to perform a satisfactory colposcopy

**Actions Prior to Procedure:**
1. Perform colposcopy with multiple directed biopsies of the cervix
2. Perform vaginal inspection with biopsy if indicated

**Contraindications:**
1. Known invasive carcinoma of cervix beyond micro invasion
2. Acute pelvic inflammatory disease or cervical culture positive for gonorrhea or chlamydia

Unless otherwise stated, **each** numbered and lettered item (except contraindications) **must** be present.

May 1989

**Procedure:** Cone biopsy of cervix, therapeutic (67.2)

**Indication:** Cervical intraepithelial neoplasia (233.1, 622.1)

**Confirmation of Indication:**
Demonstration (by exocervical or endocervical biopsies) of cervical intraepithelial neoplasia without invasion

**Actions Prior to Procedure:**
1. Perform colposcopy with multiple directed biopsies of the cervix
2. Perform vaginal inspection and biopsy if indicated

**Contraindications:**
1. Invasive carcinoma of cervix
2. Acute pelvic inflammatory disease or cervical culture positive for gonorrhea or chlamydia

Unless otherwise stated, **each** numbered and lettered item (except contraindications) **must** be present.

May 1989

**Procedure:** Surgery for stress urinary incontinence, including
1. Retropubic procedures (59.5)
2. Needle suspensions (59.6)
3. Urethral plication (59.3, 59.7 all)
4. Sling procedures (59.4)

**Indication:** Stress urinary incontinence (625.6)

**Confirmation of Indication:**
1. History of involuntary loss of urine with increased intraabdominal pressure in the absence of bladder contractions
2. Some evidence of urethral descent (eg, Q-tip, visual) on physical examination, with observation of other factors often associated with stress incontinence (eg, cystocele, rectocele, hypoestrogenism)
3. Demonstration of involuntary loss of urine

**Actions Prior to Procedure*:**
1. Obtain cystometrogram
2. Obtain urinalysis and culture

**Contraindications:**
1. Urinary tract infection
2. Neurologic cause of incontinence
3. Fistulas

*Additional procedures that may be helpful in making the diagnosis include cystourethroscopy, diary of urinary pattern, and urethral pressure profile.

Unless otherwise stated, **each** numbered and lettered item (except contraindications) **must** be present.

May 1989

**Procedure:** Oophorectomy, unilateral (65.3), or ovarian cystectomy (65.29)*

**Indication:** Asymptomatic ovarian cyst in women of reproductive age (220, 620 all)

**Confirmation of Indication:**
Presence of 1 or 2 or 3
1. Pelvic examination finding of cystic mass that is 8 cm or larger
2. Persistence of a 6–8-cm mass for two cycles
3. Presence of cystic mass that is multilocular or has solid components, as confirmed by ultrasound examination

**Actions Prior to Procedure:**
Perform vaginal examination no more than 24 hours before procedure to confirm persistence of mass

---

* Evaluation of the quality of care provided with this procedure, when performed for the indication listed, will be possible through "trending." See the discussion of trending in chapter 1.

Unless otherwise stated, **each** numbered item **must** be present.

May 1989

# chapter 4
# Administrative Organization of Quality Assurance Activities

**HOSPITAL-WIDE QUALITY ASSURANCE PROGRAM**

The hospital's governing body, administration, and medical staff share responsibility for ensuring that the health care provided by their facility is of good quality. Responsibilities should be clearly delineated, with flow of information and reporting structured to support these responsibilities.

**Responsibilities of the Medical Staff**

Through its organization into categories, departments, services, or committees, the hospital medical staff is responsible for determining criteria for membership and making recommendations to the hospital's governing body for granting initial privileges and delineating the level or category of care and, sometimes, the specific procedures that can be performed by each member of the medical staff. The medical staff also evaluates the clinical performance of all individuals with delineated privileges, monitors and evaluates the quality and appropriateness of patient care throughout the hospital, pursues opportunities to improve care, and resolves identified problems. In addition, the medical staff must have, if not total, at least shared responsibility (with the administration) for the quality assurance monitoring of nondepartmentalized functions and services, such as radiology, pathology, emergency room, ambulatory care, medical laboratory, pharmacy, and respiratory care. If appropriate, the medical staff may delegate these responsibilities to the various department or service chairpersons and to the medical directors of the various ancillary services with the stipulation that they report their activities within these areas, on a timely basis, to the quality assurance committee.

Finally, the medical staff is responsible for considering relevant findings from quality assurance activities during the process of reappraisal and renewal or revision of the clinical privileges of individual members of the medical staff.

**Responsibilities of the Hospital Administration**

The hospital administration should encourage and facilitate appropriate quality assurance activity throughout the hospital by providing the necessary personnel, space, equipment, supplies, and educational opportunities. The medical staff should regularly report quality assurance information to the hospital administration and the governing body, which are mutually responsible for the oversight of the quality assurance program. Through its administrative and supervisory staffs, the administration is also responsible for monitoring and evaluating the quality of patient care provided by health care workers who are not members of the medical staff. The administrative staff is responsible for providing a quality assurance coordinator to act as the administrative director of the hospital-wide quality assurance program.

**Hospital-wide Quality Assurance Committee**

A general hospital quality assurance committee, with the quality assurance coordinator as its administrative head, is the principal focus for quality assurance activity. This committee is responsible for overseeing the quality assurance program, for evaluating and reevaluating the various components at least annually, and for molding those components into a cohesive and functional whole. The committee should ensure that all monitoring and evaluating activities are appropriate and are effectively performed, documented, and reported. A written organization-wide plan for quality assurance is required of hospitals seeking accreditation from the Joint Commission on the Accreditation of Healthcare Organizations (the Joint Commission).

The quality assurance committee should receive and act on monthly or quarterly reports from the various entities, including department-specific quality assurance committees. The hospital-wide quality assurance committee is responsible for evaluating the effectiveness of each component of the institution's quality assurance program and, if any component is found to be less than acceptable, for recommending and overseeing such changes as are required to make the program effective. In addition, the committee tracks problems from identification to improvement or resolution and helps detect trends or patterns that involve more than one department or service.

The quality assurance committee is responsible for reporting, through the executive committee and the administration, to the hospital's governing body on the effectiveness of the hospital-wide quality assurance program. Not only does the committee communicate information concerning problems, but also it notes opportunities

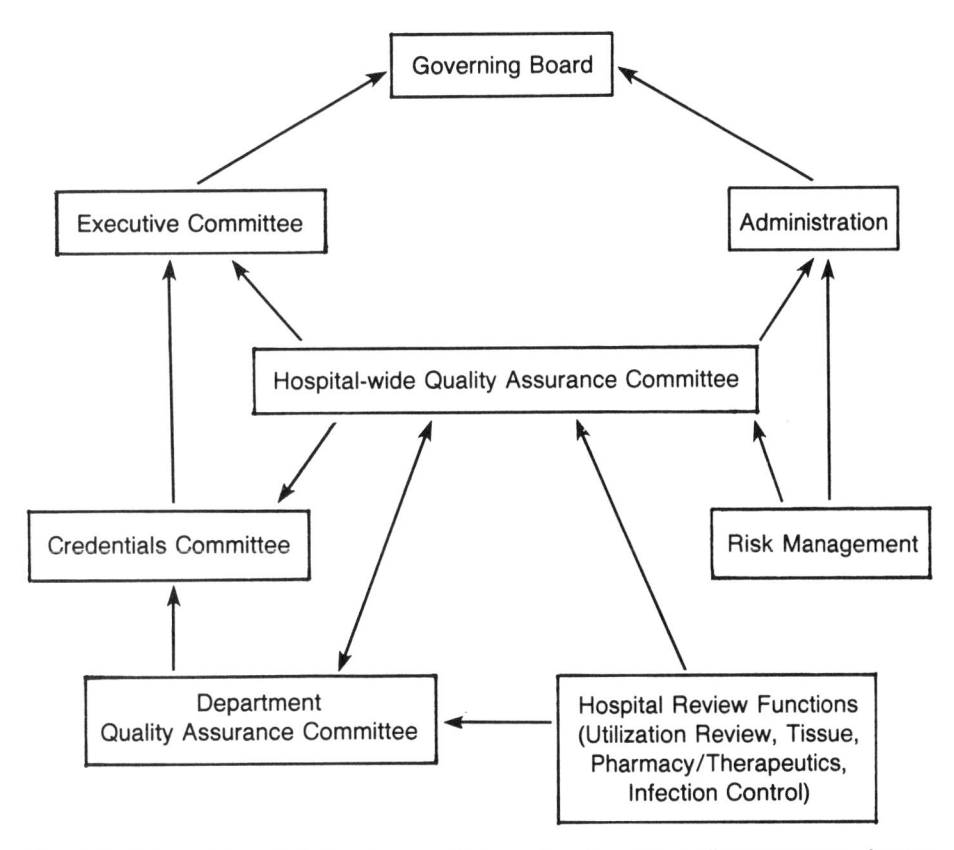

**Fig. 4-1.** A typical hospital structure and information flow for quality assurance. Arrows represent movement of information. (Source: ACOG Task Force on Quality Assurance.)

to improve patient care within the individual departments or services. Figure 4-1 illustrates one example of how quality assurance information may flow within a hospital.

## DEPARTMENT QUALITY ASSURANCE PROGRAM

### Responsibility

Individual departments also address quality issues. In hospitals that are departmentalized, the unique characteristics of the various specialties make it wise for each department of the medical staff to have a department quality assurance committee. The appropriate size and scope of each department committee depend on the size of the department itself.

In small hospitals, where each specialty may not be departmentalized, the hospital-wide quality assurance committee may monitor the quality assurance activities specific to obstetrics and gynecology. A larger hospital with a small department may have a quality assurance committee made up of three or four physicians who monitor all the quality assurance activities of the department. Major departments that provide a much broader scale of obstetric and gynecologic services may have a very large committee, consisting of representatives from the various subspecialties. In this case, several subcommittees, such as a surgical case review committee, perinatal review committee, and a credentialing committee, may perform quality assurance functions most efficiently.

**Implementation and Functioning**

The quality assurance standards of the Joint Commission emphasize the importance of planned, systematic, and ongoing monitoring and evaluation activities, as well as the need for a framework within which to conduct those activities. The Joint Commission standards set forth seven necessary characteristics of department monitoring and evaluation activities; these activities

1. Are planned, systematic, and ongoing
2. Are comprehensive
3. Are based on *indicators* and *criteria* that the department or service staff agree on and that are acceptable to the organization
4. Are accomplished by the routine collection and periodic evaluation of data
5. Result in appropriate actions to solve identified problems or identified opportunities to improve patient care
6. Are continual, in an effort to ensure that improvements in care and performance are sustained
7. Are integrated—the information derived from department monitoring and evaluation activities is shared with other departments and services and is merged, as appropriate, with information obtained throughout the organization

Elements of the Joint Commission's model for monitoring and evaluating the quality of care provided by health care organizations have been modified in this manual to demonstrate quality assurance activities at the department level. (Also see appendix A for a brief overview of the Joint Commission's Agenda for Change.)

*Assigning responsibility*

In departmentalized hospitals, the head of each department is responsible for quality assurance activities. This person identifies and assigns monitoring and evaluation responsibilities to others in the department and ensures that these responsibilities are fulfilled. Although not always necessary, a written department quality assurance plan is advisable, as department heads often find that a working outline of the department monitoring and evaluation process provides focus and direction for department quality assurance activities. Additionally, the Joint Commission requires that monthly department or service meetings be held to analyze findings related to quality of patient care.

*Identifying clinical indicators*

As discussed in chapter 2, a clinical indicator is a defined, measurable dimension of an important aspect of patient care. It describes a quantifiable clinical event, complication, or outcome for which data should be collected. Together, the staff members charged with responsibility for department quality assurance activities should formulate a list of clinical indicators to be used in monitoring the care provided in the department. A good starting point would be to review the events listed as clinical indicators in chapter 2. Staff members may also elect to create other indicators that they believe to be useful in evaluating their department's care. After formulating a list of clinical indicators, this group should present the list to the entire staff of the department of obstetrics and gynecology for refinement and approval.

*Establishing criteria sets*

Each criterion used by the department to monitor the quality of patient care should be viewed as a point on a yardstick or gauge that defines what the department considers an acceptable level of performance. Criteria sets establish a minimum standard below which care is unacceptable.

Criteria sets pertaining to patient care should be derived from authoritative sources and should be supported by the best available clinical and quality assurance literature. The criteria should be selected, developed, and adapted by staff members who are expert in the particular clinical area. Once drafted, criteria must be approved by the members of the department or service as a whole.

Chapter 3 contains a number of suggested criteria sets that may be used in assessing the appropriateness of care provided to patients by individual department members and by the department as a whole. For example, the criteria sets may be used 1) for peer review of charts identified by the clinical indicators or by other hospital reviews, such as that performed by the infection control committee; 2) for review of the appropriateness of surgery by the department quality assurance committee or by the hospital-wide surgical case review committee; or 3) in focused audits of an individual practitioner or of the entire department.

The criteria sets in chapter 3 of this manual have been reviewed by practice committees and commissions of the American College of Obstetrics and Gynecology (ACOG) and are intended to serve as a minimum standard for departments of obstetrics and gynecology that are establishing their own criteria sets. Many departments will establish more stringent criteria for some procedures, if local staffing and equipment resources permit. No department of obstetrics and gynecology should use criteria that are less stringent.

*Evaluating appropriateness of surgery*

Evaluation of the appropriateness of surgery performed by practitioners within the department of obstetrics and gynecology should be an integral part of the quality assurance program. The clinical indicators suggested in chapter 2 measure primarily patient outcomes or occurrences and are not designed to assess appropriateness in most instances. Joint Commission standards logically require hospital departments that provide surgical care to conduct a monthly surgical case review. In large departments, a surgical case review committee or the department quality assurance committee best performs this function. In hospitals with small departments, a medical staff committee may perform this task.

Currently, the Joint Commission requires that each surgical case be reviewed. When surgical case review consistently affirms the reasonableness of individual surgical procedures or the competence of individual practitioners, however, it is acceptable for subsequent reviews to focus on an adequate sample of cases. All cases in which there is a major discrepancy between preoperative and postoperative diagnosis should be evaluated.

Ideally, predetermined criteria such as those suggested in chapter 3 should be used to review surgical cases. The department may instruct the medical records abstractor to exclude from review all cases that meet the predetermined criteria, thus eliminating unnecessary and time-consuming physician case review. (See chapter 2 for suggestions regarding the implementation of such a system.)

Patterns can reveal much about the appropriateness of care. Practice variations and deficiencies become more obvious when similar types of cases are reviewed over time and across all providers. It is also important to compare the volume of cases and the complications associated with them. Insufficient justification for surgery, for example, becomes a valid measure of the appropriateness of care when analysis identifies a trend in care. This is particularly obvious if one physician performed a number of the unjustified surgical procedures.

Those variations that represent inadequate judgment, skill, or performance should be classified as deficiencies in care. When a deficiency in care is serious or widespread, there is a problem. When the quality of care is acceptable but, given the resources available, could be better, there is an opportunity for improvement.

Although some variations can be justified during the peer review process, an effectively designed and implemented quality assurance program identifies problems in care. Routine justification of all variations is inconsistent with the goal of professional self-improvement and suggests that the quality assurance program is not effective.

*Collecting and analyzing data*

There are two primary methods of data collection: the concurrent method, in which data are collected while care is being provided, and the retrospective method, in which data are collected after the care has been completed or after the patient has been discharged. Although concurrent data are particularly useful for risk management, immediate data retrieval requires a sophisticated network that may not prove practical for the assessment of the quality of care provided within a department. Retrospective data retrieval is more commonly used for reasons of simplicity and efficient utilization of staff.

A common method of retrospective data retrieval is to record data in logs placed in the various areas of the hospital used by members of the department of obstetrics and gynecology, such as the operating room, the labor and delivery rooms, and the nursery. Logs have been found to be inefficient in many circumstances, however, because their usefulness depends on the accuracy and completeness of the entries, which require cooperation of many members of the hospital staff. For this reason, chart analysis at the time of discharge seems to be the most accurate method of data retrieval. In order for this method to be effective, a trained data abstractor should review the charts of all patients discharged from the department of obstetrics and gynecology and use the clinical indicators to identify cases that require further assessment by the department's quality assurance committee. In departments of small to moderate size, a member of the hospital quality assurance department or department of medical records is generally responsible for the abstraction process. Larger departments may have the resources to retain a data abstractor to perform this task.

At regular, specified times determined by the volume of patients, services, or procedures being monitored and the importance of the indicators being monitored, the collected data should be tabulated and prepared for review by the quality assurance committee. Peer review should then be used to investigate further the variations identified and to determine whether the variations are acceptable or whether they reveal a problem. Reports from hospital-wide committees, such as the surgical case review or blood utilization committees, are also reviewed by the quality assurance committee. The results of these reviews are integrated into a comprehensive overview of department and individual physicians' practices.

Data collected over time from a number of sources are the components of individual and department data summaries. (See examples of appropriate forms in appendices B-3 through B-6.) The head of the department should examine such summaries on a quarterly basis. On at least an annual basis, pertinent physician-specific data that reflect practice quality should be incorporated into each practitioner's performance profile.

*Taking action to resolve problems*

If data analysis shows that the care provided meets the criteria and is acceptable, the monitoring and evaluating process should continue. When data analysis identifies an area of concern, a specific problem, or an opportunity to improve care or performance, a plan should be formulated to deal with the situation. Corrective action is then initiated (see chapter 5). A record should be maintained of all actions taken when problems or opportunities for improvement are identified. If a needed action exceeds the authority of the department head, he or she forwards recommendations to the body that has the authority to act. Defects in systems can be addressed by changing policies and procedures, redistributing staff, altering use of equipment and supplies, and correcting any communication problems. Findings, both good and bad, regarding the department's quality of care as identified by the department quality review process should be expeditiously reported to the hospital-wide quality assurance committee.

*Assessing actions and documenting improvement*

After enough time has elapsed for change to occur, a follow-up assessment, generally employing the same monitoring and evaluation activities that originally identified the problem, is conducted to determine whether the corrective action has resolved the problem and improved patient care and services. Initially, the follow-up assessment should focus on the problem or opportunity for improvement, not on the action taken. Monitoring and evaluation activities should continue to ensure that the problem has been permanently solved. Like the corrective action itself, the results of follow-up monitoring and evaluation activities also should be documented to provide a record of the effectiveness of the action taken.

If remedial action does not improve the quality and appropriateness of care, the problem and its potential solutions should be reassessed. A new solution should be attempted and, once again, the problem should be evaluated. Resolution of the identified problem or an improvement in care should not necessarily result in the elimination of that particular monitoring and evaluation activity; the monitoring and evaluation process should be used to maintain or improve further the quality and appropriateness of care and services.

*Incorporating relevant information into the recredentialing process*

Little is gained if an efficiently designed data retrieval process only generates data on the quality of care provided, but fails to incorporate that data into a program for the periodic reappraisal of both individual physician performance and department performance. The department's system of quality assurance should permit an evaluation of the professional performance, knowledge, judgment, and clinical or technical skills of each staff member who has privileges within the department. A form should be used to summarize the quality assurance committee's evaluation of the variations identified. (See appendix B-8 for an example.) Relevant findings from this monitoring system should be used in the reappraisal-reappointment process, including the granting or continuation of specific clinical privileges within the department.

Each physician's confidential file should contain the cumulative results of those practice variations identified as deficiencies in care by the quality assurance program. The physician's confidential file should also contain the cumulative results of other hospital-wide reviews, such as medical records review, blood utilization review, and pharmacy and therapeutic review. The combined result of reviews should be incorporated into a practitioner performance profile (see appendices B-9 and B-10).

Clinical indicator data collection forms (see appendices B-1 and B-2) should be used to collect cumulative outcome data for all cases managed by an individual physician during the course of one year. The department quality assurance committee should oversee the creation of statistical data summaries for the department as a whole and for each physician (see appendices B-3 through B-6); these data show the annual and quarterly volume of several important obstetric and gynecologic procedures. The percentage of deficiencies compared to the overall volume of care rendered by the physician should then be calculated. This type of data allows the department head or credentialing committee to compare each physician's performance with the department average for each type of service provided.

When the periodic recredentialing process has been completed, the head of the department of obstetrics and gynecology or the chairperson of the department's recredentialing committee should place in the physician's file a signed statement, noting that the full range of privileges previously granted to the individual department member has been reviewed and specifying which privileges have been recommended for continuation or restriction.

### Addressing quality assurance problems in ancillary services

On occasion, the department quality assurance committee may identify recurrent problems caused by substandard activity within ancillary services (eg, laboratory, pharmacy). Substandard practices within these areas can significantly affect the quality of care administered by the department of obstetrics and gynecology. For example, problems may arise from inadequate staffing or educational levels within the laboratory. Whenever problems of this nature occur, written requests for corrective action should be submitted to the director of the support service in question. Representatives of the department of obstetrics and gynecology should meet with the director of the support service to design and implement a corrective program. A procedure for reassessment should be designed to ensure that the problem has been resolved.

### Protection for peer review activities

To encourage self-policing by physicians, both federal and state laws provide some protection for physician peer review. The Health Care Quality Improvement Act, passed by Congress in October 1986, grants immunity from damages under federal and state laws (including antitrust provisions) to health care providers engaged in good faith peer review. (A brief overview of the important provisions of this federal legislation is included in chapter 5; complete wording of the amended law is contained in appendix D.) The majority of states have also adopted laws to encourage and protect physician peer review, although the type of immunity offered and the class of persons protected from personal liability for participating in peer review vary significantly from state to state.

Most states safeguard the confidentiality of records that are used in a quality assurance peer review action. The extent of the protection varies from jurisdiction to jurisdiction, however, and anyone engaged in peer review should know the laws of his or her state. For example, some states recognize confidentiality only for the records of a hospital review committee, while others protect all information given to the committee. In some states, the information is not admissible as evidence in a trial, but may be discoverable in pretrial proceedings. To ensure maximum protection of records, those formulating a hospital's quality review program should seek legal advice.

### Maintaining confidentiality

An evaluation of the quality and appropriateness of care, by its very nature, often involves the examination and assessment of extremely sensitive clinical material. It is important that the quality assurance program have written safeguards to ensure as much confidentiality as possible within the program.

Each practitioner within the department should be assigned a code number. On material summarized by abstractors and prepared for committee review, patients' hospital numbers and practitioners' quality assurance numbers should be used instead of their names. Likewise, numbers rather than names should be used in discussions within the committee. The codes should be broken by the department head only when necessary to act on relevant information or to continue with the recredentialing process. The use of code numbers during committee review also helps to eliminate any bias that may be present when the practitioner's name is used during the discussion and disposition of cases under review. Written materials associated with peer review, including data retrieval sheets, work forms, and minutes of meetings, should not be mailed to committee members prior to meetings. Also, this type of information should be left in the meeting room after a committee meeting and collected at the end of the meeting by specified personnel. Materials should be stamped "confidential." A patient's medical record is usually admissible in a court of law, but quality assurance documents (which should be marked as such) often are not.

A practitioner's confidential quality assurance file should be identified by a quality assurance code number only and should be maintained under lock and key in a secured area. Access to this file should be limited to those individuals with a need to know—usually the chief of staff, the department head, credentials committee chairperson, quality assurance coordinator or the quality assurance committee chairperson, and perhaps the hospital administrator and chairperson of the governing body. Individuals authorized to examine these files should be specified in the written quality assurance plan for the hospital or the department. Each physician should be guaranteed the right to review his or her file on a regular basis and respond to the information entered and stored there.

Committee members, medical record abstractors, and members of the quality assurance staff should be reminded frequently that quality assurance material is very sensitive and that such information should not be discussed openly, either inside or outside the hospital.

## NARRATIVE EXAMPLES ILLUSTRATING POSSIBLE SOURCES OF QUALITY ASSURANCE DATA

**Example 1:** Obstetric Clinical Indicators and Practitioner Performance Profile

**Example 2:** Gynecologic Clinical Indicators and Practitioner Performance Profile

**Example 3:** Infectious Disease Committee Report and Obstetric Clinical Indicators (Physician-Specific Statistics and Department Data Summary)

**Example 4:** Report from Surgical Case Review Committee

**Example 5:** Practitioner-Specific Data Summary and Surgical Case Review Committee Report

**Example 6:** Obstetric Clinical Indicators (Practitioner-Specific Statistics and Department Data Summary), Practitioner Performance Profile, and Transfusion Committee Report

## Example 1: Obstetric Clinical Indicators and Practitioner Performance Profile

The department quality assurance committee reviewed an obstetric case of practitioner 35. Care had been flagged for committee review by the clinical indicator "Birth trauma" (Ob 23). Chart review identified this complication, a depressed skull fracture of the neonate, and showed that it resulted from repeated attempts at forceps delivery. The committee judged care to be below standard. A review of the practitioner's performance profile revealed that the incidence of birth trauma among the infants whom he delivered was three times the hospital average.

The committee's findings were conveyed to the department head for possible corrective action. The confidential files showed that the department head had previously counseled practitioner 35 regarding the high rate of newborn injury during deliveries of his patients and had recommended specific educational activity. At this time, the department head recommended revocation of the obstetric privileges of practitioner 35. The case was referred to the hospital executive committee for corrective action.

NARRATIVE EXAMPLES

**Example 2: Gynecologic Clinical Indicators and Practitioner Performance Profile**

The department quality assurance committee reviewed a case in which practitioner 68 had performed gynecologic surgery. The case was identified by clinical indicator "Unplanned return to operating room for surgery during same admission" (Gyn 6). Case review revealed that the patient had been returned to the operating room following a hysterectomy because of excessive vaginal bleeding. A bleeding vaginal cuff vessel was identified and sutured. Review of the practitioner's performance profile revealed no trend of similar cases or other surgical complications. No immediate action was necessary. The case was routinely recorded in the physician's performance profile.

**Example 3: Infectious Disease Committee Report and Obstetric Clinical Indicators (Physician-Specific Statistics and Department Data Summary)**

The infectious disease committee sent a letter to the director of the obstetrics and gynecology department because the committee had noticed an increase in the incidence of wound infection in obstetric patients. The department quality assurance committee decided to collect data on the variation identified (ie, too many wound infections).

Through use of the Obstetric Clinical Indicators, patients with wound infections should have already been identified. They may have been identified by clinical indicators Ob 2, 4, or 7.

Threshold criteria were set, and the target number of wound infections (ie, the acceptable level) was determined to be zero. This number was established by staff members on the quality assurance committee and was approved by all members of the department of obstetrics and gynecology.

Data on the incidence of wound infections were collected both for the department as a whole and for individual physicians. The percentage of infections (in all deliveries) was determined for each physician. The data, collected retrospectively for the past year and divided into four quarters, were analyzed to determine whether there had actually been a recent increase in wound infections. It was determined from the data that there had been, in fact, an increase in the rate of wound infections over the past 6 months and that the incidence of wound infection among a new staff member's patients was four times that among any other staff member's patients.

Two members of the quality assurance committee of the department were assigned to scrub with the new physician to determine whether breaks in sterile technique or other factors were responsible for the infection rate among his patients. Errors in surgical technique were identified, and suggestions for correcting the deficiencies were offered to the new physician. He was informed that another audit of wound infections would be conducted in 6 months.

NARRATIVE EXAMPLES

**Example 4: Report from Surgical Case Review Committee**

Practitioner 42 performed three hysterectomies for abnormal uterine bleeding with pathologic findings of uterine polyps 2–4 cm in size. Hospital and office records of the examination, workup, and surgery for the three procedures were reviewed by means of the criteria set "Hysterectomy, abdominal or vaginal, for abnormal uterine bleeding." Findings revealed that all patients had undergone endometrial sampling procedures and had showed no evidence of neoplasia.

One patient had not undergone dilation and curettage (D&C), but had a "negative" hysteroscopy. Two patients had undergone a D&C, but minimal tissue had been obtained. There was no mention of the use of polyp forceps in either case. The department head discussed the findings of the reviews with practitioner 42. Also discussed with practitioner 42 were 1) the procedure for hysteroscopy (eg, techniques), 2) the utilization of polyp forceps at the time of a D&C, and 3) the necessity of performing a thorough D&C.

This physician's performance will be closely monitored. If there is a recurrence of the same problem, corrective action is likely to include intensive counseling with possible suspension of operating room privileges and referral to the hospital executive committee.

### Example 5: Practitioner-Specific Data Summary and Surgical Case Review Committee Report

Through the department's year-to-date data in the practitioner-specific data summaries, the quality assurance committee found that practitioner 33 had performed five hysterectomies for chronic pelvic pain, compared to a maximum of one procedure for this indication by other physicians in the department. Using the criteria set "Hysterectomy, abdominal or vaginal, for chronic pelvic pain in the absence of significant pathology," a member of the department's quality assurance committee evaluated these five charts. It was found that none of the patients had undergone a prior diagnostic laparoscopy and that two patients had experienced pain for only 3 months prior to surgery. Nonsteroidal treatment had been tried, but none of the patients had responded to the antiinflammatory drugs.

Preoperative evaluations did not consistently include an examination for potential problems in the urinary, gastrointestinal, and musculoskeletal systems. Also lacking was documentation of psychosexual and psychologic evaluation by the physician or by another health care provider. Pathologic review revealed that one patient had mild adenomyosis and another patient had a 3-cm leiomyoma. All other surgical specimens were normal. Because of these findings, all cases in which practitioner 33 had performed gynecologic surgery for other indications were reviewed; except in a few minor instances, the care provided in these cases was found to be acceptable.

The department head had a discussion with practitioner 33 concerning 1) the proper preoperative evaluation of patients who have chronic pelvic pain, but do not demonstrate significant pelvic pathology; 2) the appropriate counseling of such patients; and 3) the need to attempt other forms of medical therapy. The department head documented the meeting, including the date, the individuals present, and the content of the discussion.

In reviewing data collected over the next 6 months, the quality assurance committee identified a similar case among the patients of practitioner 33. The chart was compared with the same criteria set, and the care was found to be appropriate. No further action was recommended at that time.

The hospital-wide surgical case review committee had also noted the three surgical cases in which practitioner 33 had removed a normal uterus. This committee requested a review and response by the head of the obstetrics and gynecology department. This was done as requested.

NARRATIVE EXAMPLES

**Example 6: Obstetric Clinical Indicators (Practitioner-Specific Statistics and Department Data Summary), Practitioner Performance Profile, and Transfusion Committee Report**

Patient 12345 is a 22-year-old woman, gravida 2, para 1, who had a normal spontaneous vaginal delivery of a 3,850-g female. A second-degree laceration and excessive blood loss were complications of the otherwise normal delivery by practitioner 5. A preoperative hematocrit of 39.5 vol% and postoperative hematocrit of 26.4 vol% showed a decrease in hematocrit of 13.1 vol%.

A review of all patient records flagged for obstetric clinical indicator "Excessive blood loss" revealed that 3.4% of all patients discharged from the obstetric service had experienced this complication. Over a 3-month period, records representing 7%, 8%, and 8.4%—well above the department average—of the discharged patients of practitioners 5, 6, and 7 were flagged by the screen. These physicians were advised to review their practice patterns to avoid unnecessary blood loss. During the next 3 months, the department average decreased from 3.4% to 3.1%, and the percentage of records flagged among the discharged patients of practitioners 6 and 7 decreased to 1.2% and 3%, respectively. However, 9.1% of the patients delivered by practitioner 5 during this period had a decrease in hematocrit of more than 11 vol%. Because of this continued higher-than-expected rate of blood loss, all deliveries performed by practitioner 5 were reviewed.

It was determined that the patients of practitioner 5 had more than twice the average incidence of second-degree or third-degree lacerations. The department head discussed these issues with him and advised him to adjust his practice in order to decrease the incidence of excessive blood loss among his patients. Relevant educational opportunities were suggested. Three months after these changes, the percentage of patients of practitioner 5 who experienced excessive blood loss was 3%, equal to the department average. The incidences of trauma and lacerations among his patients were also found to be average.

# chapter 5
# Corrective Action

When the department quality assurance committee identifies specific deficiencies in the quality of care, the department head (or the person designated by the hospital bylaws) should take appropriate action to correct the deficiency promptly and efficiently.

### MODIFYING CLINICAL ACTIVITY OF AN INDIVIDUAL

When a specific practitioner's performance profile indicates that he or she is practicing in a manner not in keeping with the standards of the department, the department head selects a corrective action based on the number and severity of the deficiencies identified. When uncertain as to whether corrective action is necessary, the department head may elect to observe further the practitioner's performance before intervening. If action is required, the department head may elect to counsel the practitioner informally or to discuss alternative plans of care that would have been more suitable in the cases identified as deficient. More formally, the department head may find it necessary to suggest remedial education, to require proctoring, or even to recommend restriction of the practitioner's privileges. Any recommendation for action of a serious nature should be made by the executive committee of the medical staff. Final action on the department head's recommendations for restriction of privileges is the ultimate responsibility of the hospital's governing body.

Figure 5-1 diagrams typical processes of responding to identified variations in clinical practice, whether these variations have been observed within the practice of an individual or of several members of a department.

### Discussion

The initial step in taking informal corrective action is to review with the practitioner whose performance is in question the data that suggest the deficiency or deficiencies. There may be an adequate explanation for the apparent deficiencies. In other cases,

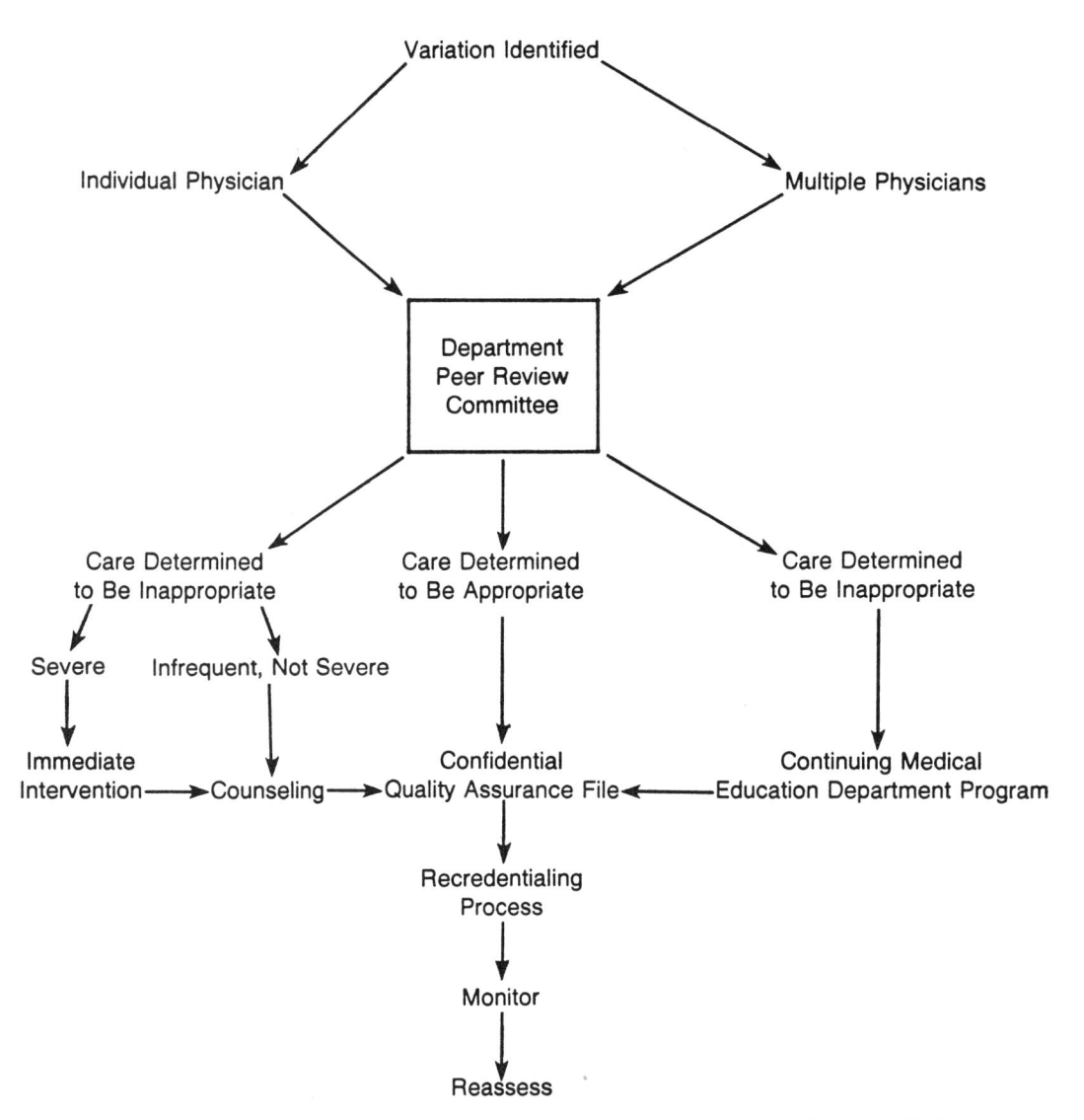

**Fig. 5-1.** Responding to variations and deficiencies in practice. (Modified from Robert N. Yelverton, MD. Reprinted with permission.)

the department head may recommend alternative treatment plans or techniques that will correct the problem. A frank discussion initiated by the department head is often very effective and may be all that is necessary to alter substandard practice.

Although a discussion of this nature is conducted informally, written documentation of the date, the individuals present, and the agreed-upon resolution of the problem is important. Without documentation of the initial, informal corrective action, the practitioner in question may subsequently challenge more formal corrective action. Bylaws regarding due process should be followed during all stages of corrective actions.

*Example:* During the course of its routine assessment of patient records by means of the clinical indicators used for department quality assurance review, the department quality assurance committee noted the records of two patients attended by practitioner 21. These two cases were flagged because of the presence of the clinical indicators "Delivery of an infant with a birth weight less than 2,500 g or respiratory distress syndrome after a planned repeat cesarean delivery, or following induction of labor" (Ob 14 and Ob 15). In both cases, practitioner 21 had performed scheduled repeat cesarean deliveries, resulting in the birth of infants who developed respiratory distress syndrome and required admission to the neonatal intensive care unit. The quality assurance committee judged that both cases involved the delivery of a preterm infant and demonstrated a deficiency in care, in that practitioner 21 had failed to document the gestational age despite preestablished criteria for such documentation. Both infants were subsequently discharged without significant sequelae.

The department head was routinely notified of the identified deficiencies in care. His review of the practitioner's performance profile revealed no similar prior deficiencies in care, and the practitioner's performance in other areas of obstetric and gynecologic care was acceptable.

The department head, along with the chairperson of the quality assurance committee, then discussed the problem with practitioner 21. The appropriate methods of determining gestational age in patients who are to undergo repeat elective cesarean deliveries were discussed. Practitioner 21 accepted these recommendations and stated that he would incorporate these standards into his clinical practice. The department head then documented the discussion and plan of action in the confidential quality assurance file of practitioner 21. Subsequent review of this practitioner's performance profile has revealed no further incidence of similar complications.

## Observation

If the deficiency identified concerns a practitioner's skills in a specific technique, the department head may elect, before taking any corrective action, to have a designated member of the department who is known to be skilled in that technique observe the practitioner's skills.

*Example:* The operating room nurse coordinator reported to the department head that practitioner 71 was performing laparoscopic examinations using techniques that, in the opinion of the operating room nursing personnel, were unconventional and might result in complications. When the department head and the quality assurance committee chairperson reviewed the practitioner's performance profile, they found no clinical indicators reflecting complications associated with this practitioner's laparoscopic procedures. The department head discussed the nurses' voiced concern with practitioner 71, who felt that his techniques were appropriate, but agreed to have a physician known to be skilled in laparoscopic procedures observe his techniques in the operating room.

The physician–observer reported that, although the techniques used by practitioner 71 to establish the pneumoperitoneum and introduce the laparoscopic trocar were somewhat different from those used by the majority of surgeons on the staff, the techniques were both acceptable and safe. No action was necessary. The review was documented and placed in the confidential quality assurance file of practitioner 71. Nursing staff was informed of the action taken.

## External Peer Review

On occasion, an identified deficiency or the standards by which a deficiency is identified are controversial, and members of the department cannot agree on the proper action to take. In these instances, the department head may elect to invite an outside consultant to review the alleged deficiency and to render an opinion.

*Example:* The hospital-wide surgical case review committee concluded, based on preestablished criteria, that practitioner 3 was performing diagnostic cone biopsies without justifiable indications. The committee noted that this practitioner had performed three excisional cone biopsies on patients with abnormal Pap smears without first performing colposcopic examinations and biopsies. The committee concluded that, if the practitioner's office evaluation of the abnormal Pap smears had been appropriate, the cone biopsies might not have been necessary.

The department head reviewed the three cases and agreed with the committee decision. When practitioner 3 was apprised of this opinion, however, he refused to accept it and stated that only a gynecologic oncologist could render an authoritative opinion. Because there was no gynecologic oncologist on the hospital staff, the department head retained a gynecologic oncologist from a nearby medical center to review the cases in question. The consultant agreed with the committee's conclusion that the cases had not been managed appropriately.

Practitioner 3 was instructed that, in the future, he should perform appropriate preliminary diagnostic procedures before performing diagnostic cone biopsy. The incident, committee report, consultant's report, and corrective action outlined by the department head were included in the practitioner's confidential quality assurance file. For the next two years, all cone biopsies performed by this practitioner were reviewed to ensure his compliance with the recommended practices.

**Remedial Education**

When an identified problem involves a lack of specific knowledge or of a specific clinical skill in a practitioner whose performance has been judged satisfactory in other areas of practice, the department head may elect to require the practitioner to complete a remedial education program designed to correct the deficiency.

*Example:* The department quality assurance committee concluded that practitioner 10 had the highest primary cesarean delivery rate in the hospital, with a disproportionate percentage of the procedures being performed for fetal distress (see glossary). After a year-long review of all the cesarean deliveries for fetal distress performed by practitioner 10, the committee concluded that 60% of these deliveries were clinically unjustified. This conclusion was based on a review of the relevant electronic fetal monitoring strips and related clinical events.

The department head was notified of the committee's conclusion, and a conference was arranged with the practitioner in question. After this conference, the department head concluded that practitioner 10 lacked a basic knowledge of fetal heart rate monitoring and had no clear understanding of the clinical findings that indicate fetal distress. The department head recommended that practitioner 10 attend a continuing medical education course in fetal monitoring. Furthermore, until the practitioner completed the course and demonstrated proficiency in interpreting fetal heart rate patterns, the department head recommended that the practitioner obtain a consultation, when possible, prior to performing a cesarean delivery for fetal distress. The physician accepted this decision.

Following completion of the course in fetal heart rate monitoring, the physician was allowed to perform cesarean deliveries for fetal distress without a consultation. All cases of cesarean delivery for fetal distress performed by practitioner 10 were monitored by the quality assurance committee for a period of 2 years.

**Proctoring**

In certain instances, the department head may decide that the interests of quality care and fairness are best served by requiring a peer to scrub and observe a practitioner on a given number of cases. Alternatively, the peer may be asked to review the charts of that practitioner's patients on a concurrent or retrospective basis to ensure that professional standards are maintained.

*Example:* The hospital-wide surgical case review committee reported to the department head that, in four recently reviewed cases of practitioner 13, there were significant discrepancies between the preoperative diagnoses and the postoperative tissue reports. In addition, practitioner 13 had performed surgery to remove simple cysts of the ovary in four cases. In the opinion of the committee and the department head, these events resulted from improper evaluation or improper therapy prior to surgery.

Practitioner 13 refused to participate in a proctoring arrangement, prompting the department head to refer the matter to the executive committee of the hospital. After review, this committee approved the recommended proctoring. Although practitioner 13 appealed the decision and was allowed to continue practicing during the appeal process, the governing body of the hospital upheld the department head's decision. The final decision of the governing body required that all cases of patients admitted for gynecologic surgery by practitioner 13 be subject to a proctor's review by a member of an appointed panel of active staff members in good standing in the department of obstetrics and gynecology. Cases are allowed to proceed to surgery only after the proctor agrees that surgery is indicated. Practitioner 13 will remain on the hospital staff with probational privileges for 2 years. After that time, active staff privileges will be restored if review of his surgical cases show no deficiency.

### Probation

Conditional privileges, pending further assessment of a practitioner's skills, may be imposed along with any of the corrective actions that have been described. The hospital's due process provisions, as specified in its bylaws, should be carefully followed.

### Limiting Privileges

With more serious deficiencies, it may be necessary to limit a practitioner's privileges (ie, to deny a practitioner the authority to perform procedures that are beyond his or her documented competence). Often, practitioners with a documented performance problem involving a particular procedure or procedures will voluntarily limit their privileges. Otherwise, formal proceedings (as prescribed in the hospital bylaws) are necessary to limit privileges.

*Example:* In its review of patient charts flagged by clinical indicators, the department quality assurance committee noted four charts of patients who had undergone laparoscopy by practitioner 4. These cases were identified for review by the clinical indicators 1) "Unplanned return to the operating room for surgery during the same admission" (Gyn 6); 2) "Unplanned removal, injury, or repair of organ during operative procedure" (Gyn 9); and 3) "Ambulatory surgery patient admitted for surgical complication" (Gyn 7). The committee reported its findings to the department head with the comment that these four cases appeared to demonstrate deficiencies in care.

The department head reviewed the practitioner's confidential quality assurance file and found that the occurrence of similar complications in the past had prompted the previous department head to suspend temporarily the laparoscopic privileges of practitioner 4 until he had completed a remedial education course in diagnostic and operative laparoscopy. Although he had completed the course, the recent complications among the laparoscopy patients of practitioner 4 also resulted from deficiencies in care. For this reason, the department head recommended that the diagnostic and operative laparoscopy privileges of practitioner 4 be permanently suspended. The hospital executive committee upheld the department head's recommendation after a thorough review. Although the practitioner challenged the executive committee's decision, the governing body of the hospital upheld the decision after an appropriate review and exhaustion of the appeal process, as outlined in the hospital bylaws. Practitioner 4 retained the remainder of his gynecologic privileges, as the hospital quality assurance monitors did not reveal any significant problems in other areas of gynecologic surgery.

### Revoking Privileges

An extreme step, the revocation of all privileges, is used only when other measures have failed or when it is necessary to ensure quality of care and to protect the safety of patients.

*Example:* After reviewing the confidential quality assurance file of practitioner 26, the hospital credentials committee recommended that the practitioner's clinical privileges be revoked. A number of incidents involving deficiencies in care had been documented. The file also contained documentation of three conferences between practitioner 26 and the head of the department, conferences that had been conducted in the hopes of improving the practitioner's clinical performance. All efforts to improve his performance, including remedial education, had failed, however. Two years before the recommendation of the credentials committee, probation and proctoring of the practitioner's gynecologic surgery cases had been instituted. Following reestablishment of full clinical privileges, screening with the clinical indicators revealed an insufficient improvement in the practitioner's performance. The hospital executive committee reviewed the credential committee's recommendations and concluded that the practitioner's privileges should be revoked. This decision was approved by the governing body of the hospital after the appropriate review had been conducted and the appeal process, as outlined in the hospital bylaws, had been followed.

**Summary Suspension**

Whenever action must be taken immediately to protect the health and welfare of patients under the care of a practitioner, most hospital bylaws give the chief of staff, the department head, or the chief administrative officer the authority to recommend summary suspension of all or any portion of a practitioner's clinical privileges. A summary suspension becomes effective immediately upon issuance. Arrangements are then made to transfer the care of the practitioner's hospitalized patients to other practitioners. Because of its obvious implications, such a step is usually taken only when, in the opinion of the officer charged with invoking such a suspension, the practitioner has become so physically or mentally impaired or his conduct so outrageous as to be an immediate threat to patients under his care. The practitioner whose privileges have been suspended is entitled to a hearing on the matter within a reasonable period of time, usually specified by the hospital bylaws.

*Example:* The department head was notified by the nurse coordinator of the labor and delivery area that practitioner 11, who had recently been granted privileges at the hospital to attend a patient in labor, was acting in a manner that suggested substance abuse.

The department head had been monitoring the practice activities of practitioner 11 closely because of a previously unconfirmed report of similar behavior in the past. After interviewing him, the department head concluded that the practitioner was indeed acting in a manner that suggested substance abuse, was mentally impaired, and appeared to be a threat to the patients under his care. When the department head directly confronted the practitioner with these suspicions, the practitioner admitted to substance abuse. The clinical privileges of practitioner 11 were summarily suspended. Hospitalized patients attended by practitioner 11 were assigned to other physicians during their hospitalization, and a hearing on the matter was scheduled for 2 weeks from the date of suspension.

## MODIFYING CLINICAL ACTIVITY OF A DEPARTMENT

Problems identified through the department's quality assurance program can be useful guides in the development of continuing medical education programs for department staff members. Often, an effective quality assurance program reveals deficiencies that involve several practitioners within the department. In these instances, the department head may elect to conduct a department-wide, focused audit, using criteria sets similar to those outlined in chapter 3, and applying these minimum standards to all department members. If the problem is found to be widespread, a problem-oriented, continuing medical education program may be the best way to bring both the deficiencies and alternative clinical approaches to the attention of all department members. If the department quality assurance program is effectively designed, continued monitoring will demonstrate the effectiveness or ineffectiveness of such an education program. Presentation of problem cases to the medical staff (without identification of either patient or practitioner) may also serve as a method of remedial education.

## DUE PROCESS

Based on provisions of the Fifth and Fourteenth Amendments to the U.S. Constitution, the principle of due process protects certain rights of individuals from state and federal action. Consequently, due process requirements as they apply to the granting of hospital privileges were thought at one time to apply only to public hospitals. State laws and judicial decisions have been extending the concept of due process rights to actions by private hospitals. The Health Care Quality Improvement Act of 1986 underscores the need for all hospitals to follow due process requirements at all stages of disciplinary proceedings. As soon as a deficiency is identified, even before official proceedings begin, it is essential to ensure fairness, impartiality, and respect for the rights of individuals.

Each hospital should have due process provisions in its bylaws. These bylaws must specify the procedures to be followed in a disciplinary or corrective action. Very basically, courts have interpreted the due process rights to include the following elements:

*Notice:* The individual practitioner affected must be given written notice of adverse action and the right to request a hearing. The notice must state the basis for the action.

*Hearing:* If requested by the affected practitioner, a hearing before an unbiased panel must be afforded within a reasonable period of time. The practitioner has a right to challenge the charges through examination of witnesses, presentation of evidence, and a written statement.

*Decision:* A final written decision must be issued.

*Appeal:* The individual should have the right to appeal the hearing committee's decision to the governing body of the hospital. The governing body's decision is final, although the individual may try to seek judicial relief.

Figure 5-2 diagrams one hearing and appeal process.

## HEALTH CARE QUALITY IMPROVEMENT ACT OF 1986

In 1986, Congress enacted the Health Care Quality Improvement Act (PL 99-660, as amended by PL 100-177; 42 USC 11101 et seq; see appendix D). One of its purposes was to encourage physician participation in quality assurance programs by conferring immunity from actions for damages under federal and state laws to those engaged in peer review of physician conduct and competence. This immunity attaches only to a peer review action taken in the reasonable belief that it is warranted, will improve the quality of health care, and is based on a reasonable fact-finding effort. The act requires "adequate notice and hearing procedures" for the physician who is the subject of the review [42 USC § 11112(a)(3)]. The initial notice of proposed action given to the physician must state the basis for the proposed action and must advise the physician of his or her right to a hearing and of the procedural hearing rights that he or she will have. At least 30 days in advance, the physician must be notified of the time and place of the hearing and must be given a list of the witnesses who will testify. The

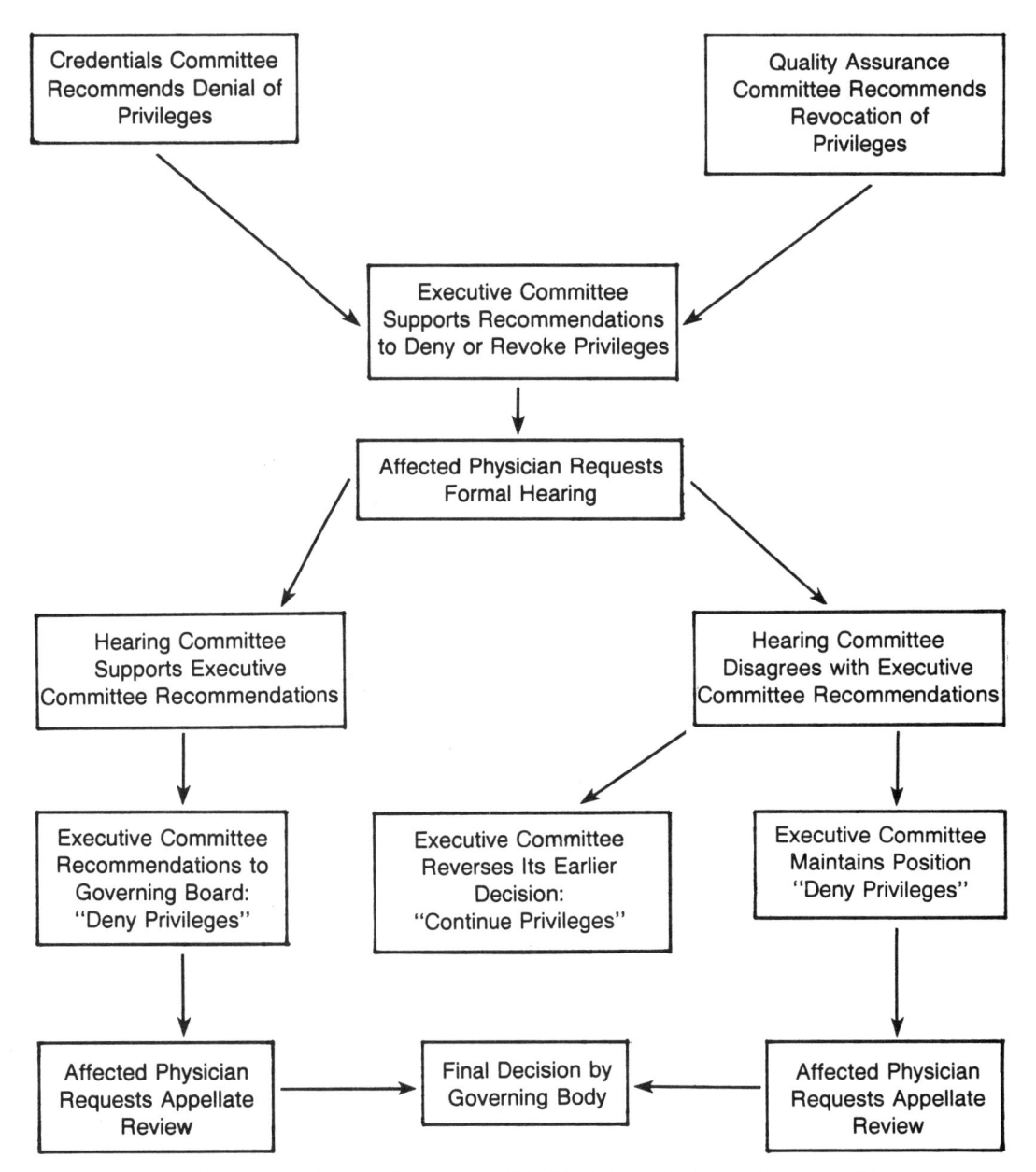

**Fig. 5-2.** Hearing and appeal process. (Modified from Bylaws, Humana Women's Hospital, Tampa, Florida. Reprinted with permission.)

hearing must be before an arbitrator, hearing officer, or panel whose members are not in "direct economic competition" with the physician who is the subject of the review [42 USC § 11112(b)].

The act [42 USC § 11112(b)(3)] also specifies the particular due process rights that a hearing must provide the physician being reviewed in order to meet the statutory requirement of "adequate notice and hearing procedures" that triggers immunity. These are the rights to

- Be represented by an attorney or other individual of his or her choice
- Receive a written record of the proceedings
- Call, examine, and cross-examine witnesses
- Present relevant evidence
- Submit a written statement

70  Quality Assurance

- Receive a copy of written recommendations of the hearing officer or panel
- Receive a copy of the written decision of the health care entity, including a statement of the basis for the decision

In its requirements for adequate notice and hearing procedures, the statute creates, in effect, a new due process standard that hospitals must follow in order to maximize protection for peer review activities.

The Health Care Quality Improvement Act of 1986 gives some leeway to hospital peer review committees in designing hearing procedures. One provision allows immunity to be given when peer review actions follow "such other procedures as are fair to the physician under the circumstances" [42 USC § 11112(a)(3)]. Thus, under the act, a hospital that does not want its peer review system to be as complex as that outlined in the act does not necessarily lose its immunity to actions for damages. In such a situation, however, the hospital still needs a written procedure that includes the rudiments of due process. The Joint Commission on the Accreditation of Healthcare Organizations guidelines and state legal requirements should always be met, at a minimum.

The immunity from federal actions for damages granted by the Health Care Quality Improvement Act of 1986 became effective in November 1986. Immunity from actions under state laws goes into effect on October 14, 1989; however, a state legislature may opt for earlier coverage under the act or may choose to opt out of the act's coverage.

## CORRECTIVE ACTION PROCESSES

Every hospital should have procedures in place for investigating possible substandard quality of care by a physician. Attention may be focused on a physician in several ways (eg, the hospital's ongoing quality assurance program, patient complaint, colleagues' observations). A hospital's bylaws may authorize the formation of a specific committee to investigate problems in the quality of care. If not, an ad hoc committee may be appointed by the medical staff and charged with the responsibility of investigating a particular problem and, if appropriate, recommending corrective actions. Many hospitals have found such a mechanism to be effective.

If the hospital uses an investigative committee to make recommendations to the "fair hearing" committee, certain guidelines should be kept in mind. The committee's membership should consist of reasonable practitioners who are not in direct personal or economic conflict with the physician being investigated. The committee should be "briefed" about its function by legal counsel or by a representative of the medical staff. The committee should assemble relevant facts and materials, interview individuals as appropriate (including the physician who is being investigated), and make a report to the body that requested the review. Any applicable bylaws must, of course, be followed.

# chapter 6
# Risk Management Through Quality Assurance

H ospitals sometimes view risk management and quality assurance programs as separate and distinct entities. Before quality assurance and risk management programs are established in any given department or hospital, the desired primary function of each activity should be clarified.

**QUALITY ASSURANCE AND RISK MANAGEMENT**

Quality assurance in a hospital setting has been defined as an effort to enhance patient care through the ongoing, objective assessment of important aspects of patient care and the correction of identified problems. Traditionally, risk management has been defined as an effort to identify, prevent, and evaluate risk, and to reduce or eliminate financial loss. Many, but not all, components of the two programs overlap. In health care, the risk of patient loss and the risk of financial loss are directly related. Events such as loss of life, surgical error, failure to diagnose correctly, unexpected adverse outcome of treatment, and birth-related injury are quality of care concerns as well as risk management issues.

An effective quality assurance program that integrates and coordinates all quality assessment activities is essential to an effective hospital risk management program. The complexity of modern medicine and medical technology has increased the chance of errors, and hospitals have come to recognize that the solution to the increased risk of liability claims as a result of such potential harm to patients is the *prevention* of liability claims. Data analysis and the resolution of problems identified through quality assurance activity, as well as liability control once injuries have occurred, are important preventive strategies.

Quality assurance and risk management programs are both designed for protection. Quality assurance focuses on the protection of patients. The diligent practice of quality care, however, also reduces the risk of ordinary negligence and protects against financial loss. Even so, risk management's focus on protecting corporate assets and thus ensuring the institution's continued financial ability to provide ongoing care to the community it serves necessitates activities beyond the scope of quality assurance. Once an adverse outcome occurs, risk management must go beyond the immediate correction of an identified problem to minimize the risk impact and protect the hospital against catastrophic losses. Table 6-1 delineates similarities and differences between quality assurance and traditional risk management.

Although their objectives are quite distinct, the degree of overlap between quality assurance and risk management is significant, and integrating the two activities to some extent is advantageous. An integrated approach can avoid duplication of effort in collecting and analyzing data. Also, the purposes and functions of quality assurance and risk management complement one another. An integrated approach to both activities establishes an optimal communication link that may provide new solutions to problems.

## INTEGRATION OF QUALITY ASSURANCE AND RISK MANAGEMENT

The department level is an ideal point at which to integrate quality assurance and risk management activities, particularly in a department of obstetrics and gynecology where exposure to liability is extremely high.

**Table 6-1.** Comparison of Quality Assurance and Traditional Risk Management

| Characteristic | Quality Assurance | Traditional Risk Management |
|---|---|---|
| Purpose | Ensure that quality of care is optimal—evaluate practitioner performance and protect patients | Minimize the hospital's losses—protect hospital |
| Character | Educational/remedial | Crisis intervention |
| Function | Measure actual care against standards; when care does not meet standards, take remedial action | Detect risks to the hospital, then prevent the recurrence or minimize their effect when they do occur |
| Patients involved | Single patient or group of patients, discharged or still hospitalized; patterns or recurrent problems in patient care are assessed | Single patient discharged or still hospitalized—isolated events |
| Time frame | Usually retrospective or concurrent with patient stay | May be concurrent or retrospective but usually coincides with awareness of potential loss |
| "Standard" | Written, explicit, clinically based criteria | Unwritten, implicit criteria (what people think is an "incident") |

A well-planned and carefully administered quality assurance program within the department of obstetrics and gynecology can assist the hospital-wide risk management program by resolving patient care problems that frequently result in liability claims. Careful analysis of cases involving birth trauma, intrapartum hypoxemia, maternal and infant mortality, and surgical complications should result in the identification and resolution of problems, thus improving the quality of patient care and reducing the risk of liability exposure of the hospital and the medical staff.

The quality assurance committee of the department of obstetrics and gynecology can also be a valuable resource for the hospital's risk management program. Unless it is inadvisable under state law, the quality assurance committee can review liability claims related to obstetric and gynecologic care and advise the hospital as to the quality of care that was provided. Review of such cases by the department quality assurance committee also allows the department to review the effectiveness of its quality assurance program, as the clinical indicators used by the department for occurrence screening should have identified the problem independent of the legal claim. If repeated claims of merit have not been identified through the existing quality assurance program, the program, particularly the clinical indicators used for screening, should be reassessed.

The department quality assurance committee is also in an ideal position to advise the department of risk management on problems in support services and equipment that affect obstetric and gynecologic care. For example, inadequate staffing of nurses in the labor and delivery area or poorly maintained laparoscopic equipment are problems that may be overlooked in the hospital-wide risk management program, but the associated risks to patients may be very apparent to the practitioners within the department of obstetrics and gynecology. A written communication to the risk management department may resolve such problems when other attempts at correction have failed.

Although the integration of quality assurance and risk management functions is logical and advisable in most situations, there are potentially negative aspects in such an integration. For example, the relative legal status of quality assurance and risk management data, such as medical audits or incident reports, vary from state to state and therefore should be researched. Reports of risk management activity may be easily accessible under the same state laws that grant immunity from discovery to medical staff peer review activities and records. Care must be taken to avoid potential problems when information is freely shared between the two groups.

## QUALITY OF MEDICAL RECORDS

One of the most effective strategies for dealing with issues of quality of health care and risk management is the establishment of a mechanism for checking the timely completion, adequacy, and accuracy of all medical records. Acceptable methods for correcting or adding supplemental information should be explained to the medical staff. Members of the staff should understand that incomplete records will result in disciplinary action.

## QUALIFICATIONS OF MEDICAL STAFF

Applicants for the medical staff should be asked to complete a written application that includes information about their mental and physical health status and any felony convictions. They should also be informed that the responsibility for timely submission of all documents of verification and reference rests with them.

Careful verification of medical staff applicants' licensure, education, clinical training, and experience are mandatory for preventing threats to quality of care and risks of liability. Contact should be made with the chairperson/director of the clinical program (the specific department or service) with which the applicant was most recently affiliated, as well as with the chief of the applicant's residency program. Reference forms should include questions about clinical competence, behavior/ethics, standing as a medical staff member of another hospital, and any practice problems that may have occurred in the past. Applicants should be tracked from medical school to the present, and any gaps should be explained. The applicant should be asked about both settled and outstanding liability claims. Courts and the Joint Commission on the Accreditation of Healthcare Organizations (the Joint Commission) have stressed the rights and duties of hospitals to verify physician-applicants' qualifications and their suitability to provide patient care. This includes the ability to work with others.

## PRIVILEGE DELINEATION

Whatever criteria are established for the delineation of privileges must be relevant, fair, and applied to all applicants and staff members. Training, experience, and current competence must ultimately be the bases for the granting and renewing of privileges. A critical step prior to granting or renewing privileges is to review quality assurance information, which should provide insights into practitioners' competence and medical judgment. Board certification is an insufficient criterion upon which to admit a physician to the medical staff or to grant privileges.

There are at least three primary methods of classifying clinical privileges:

1. By checklists (eg, illnesses, procedures)
2. Grouped by medical specialty or body systems
3. By categories based on degree of case complexity and physician qualifications

Categorization may be the most comprehensive means of delineating privileges. Neither ACOG nor the Joint Commission dictate which method hospitals should use. Staff members should reapply for specific clinical privileges at the time of recredentialing (at least biennially). Privileges requested for performance of procedures within each specialty are recommended by the heads of the respective departments.

# Appendices

# Appendix A
# The Joint Commission's Agenda for Change

In the fall of 1986, the Joint Commission on the Accreditation of Healthcare Organizations (the Joint Commission) launched a major developmental project entitled the Agenda for Change. The goal of the program is to develop an outcome-oriented monitoring and evaluation process that will assist health care organizations in improving the quality of care that they provide. As early as 1990, hospitals accredited by the Joint Commission will begin to participate in the new monitoring, survey, and accreditation process.

The Joint Commission has also planned other activities, such as:

- A communication effort to maintain and enhance Joint Commission relationships with provider health care organizations and professionals while fostering broader relationships with the government, business, labor, insurance, and consumer communities
- An educational effort to expand and improve Joint Commission educational and technical assistance services

Through the Agenda for Change, the Joint Commission intends to modify its standards, as well as its survey and monitoring processes, in ways that will make its accreditation decisions as accurate and meaningful as possible. The project is specifically designed to increase the clinical focus of the quality-related activities in the organization and to stress the importance of performance outcomes, both organizational and clinical.

The new monitoring and evaluation process will have three major components:

1. The use of severity-adjusted measurement of clinical indicators to obtain a better analysis of the organization's provision of care to patients and the identification of organizational management activities that directly affect the quality of care
2. Modification of the survey and monitoring process from one that relies only on triennial on-site visits and focused contingencies to one that involves periodic surveys supported by an ongoing data collection and analysis system with continuous feedback to organizations about their performance
3. Accreditation decisions that are based on the effectiveness of an organization's attention to possible quality of care problems and standards that are closely related to organizational effectiveness

The Joint Commission will introduce clinical indicators that reflect important dimensions of care and address high-volume, high-risk, or problem areas of clinical practice. These indicators will focus on both organization-wide and specialty-specific issues.

The indicators will be used to monitor diagnostic and treatment activities related to the structure, process, or outcome of care. Clinical indicators are not meant to be used as direct measurements of quality; they are simply "flags" to identify potential problems that warrant further review. The institution's own peer review and problem analysis processes remain the foundation of effective quality assessment and the focus of Joint Commission accreditation.

The Joint Commission intends to pool clinical indicator data collected by organizations so that an individual facility can compare itself to similar institutions. Because not every health care organization treats the same kind of patient, some form of case mix/severity adjustment will be used to help ensure that the groups being compared are reasonably similar.

The Joint Commission is also establishing liaison relationships with clinical groups that are developing indicators and plans to draw upon the efforts of those groups when they relate to project activities. It is felt that these new initiatives will place the Joint Commission in a far more supportive role in helping health care organizations make better decisions based on better information.

# Appendix B
# Sample Data Collection Forms

## Appendix B-1
## Sample Data Collection Form: Obstetric Clinical Indicators*

Mother _____ Hosp. # _____ Disch Date _____
Baby _____ Hosp. # _____ Disch Date _____
Del Date _____ MD Code # _____
Apgar at 5 minutes _____ Apgar at 10 minutes _____
Birth weight (g) _____ Gestational age _____
Adm Hct _____ Hb _____ Lowest Hct _____ Hb _____
Major congenital anomalies _____
Repeat C/S _____ Primary C/S _____

**A. Maternal Indicators**

1. Maternal mortality — Y N
2. Unplanned readmission within 14 days — Y N
3. Cardiopulmonary arrest — Y N
4. In-hospital initiation of antibiotics 24 hours or more following term vaginal delivery — Y N
5. Unplanned removal, injury, or repair of organ during operative procedure — Y N
6. In-hospital maternal red blood cell transfusion or hematocrit of less than 22 vol% or hemoglobin less than 7.0 g or decrease in hematocrit of 11 vol% or hemoglobin of 3.5 g or more — Y N
7. Maternal length of stay more than 5 days after vaginal delivery or more than 7 days after cesarean delivery — Y N
8. Eclampsia — Y N
9. Delivery unattended by the "responsible physician" — Y N
10. Postpartum return to delivery room or operating room for management — Y N
11. Induction of labor for an indication other than diabetes, premature rupture of membranes, pregnancy-induced hypertension, postterm gestation, intrauterine growth retardation, cardiac disease, isoimmunization, fetal demise, or chorioamnionitis — Y N
    a. Cesarean delivery required — Y N
12. Primary cesarean delivery for fetal distress — Y N
13. Primary cesarean delivery for failure to progress — Y N
14. Delivery of an infant with a birth weight less than 2,500 g or respiratory distress syndrome after planned repeat cesarean delivery — Y N
15. Delivery of an infant with a birth weight less than 2,500 g or respiratory distress syndrome following induction of labor — Y N

---

* The presence in a patient's medical record of any item on this list will be indicated by a circled "Y." This in turn will cause the patient's record to be flagged for evaluation by a physician. (Modified from a form developed by C. Irving Meeker, MD, for use at Maine Medical Center, Portland, Maine. Reprinted with permission.)

**B. Neonatal Indicators**

16. Perinatal mortality of a fetus or infant surviving less than 28 days and weighing 500 g or more at delivery — Y  N
17. Intrapartum death, in-hospital, of a fetus weighing 500 g or more — Y  N
18. Neonatal mortality of an inborn infant with a birth weight of 750–999 g in an institution with a neonatal intensive care unit (NICU) — Y  N
19. Delivery of an infant weighing less than 1,800 g in an institution without an NICU — Y  N
20. Transfer of a neonate to an NICU in another institution — Y  N
21. Term infant admitted to an NICU — Y  N
22. Apgar score of 4 or less at 5 minutes — Y  N
23. Birth trauma (#767 in ICD-9-CM directory), such as shoulder dystocia, cephalohematoma, Erb palsy, and clavicular fracture, but not caput — Y  N
24. Diagnosis of fetal "massive aspiration syndrome" (#770.1 in ICD-9-CM) — Y  N
25. Inborn term infant with clinically apparent seizures recorded prior to discharge — Y  N

# Appendix B-2
# Sample Data Collection Form: Gynecologic Clinical Indicators*

Patient _____ Hosp. # _____ Disch Date _____
Date of Surgery _____ MD Code # _____
Adm Hct _____ Hb _____ Lowest Hct _____ Hb _____

| | | | |
|---|---|---|---|
| 1. | Unplanned readmission within 14 days | Y | N |
| 2. | Admission after a return visit to the emergency room for the same problem | Y | N |
| 3. | Cardiopulmonary arrest | Y | N |
| 4. | Occurrence of an infection not present on admission | Y | N |
| 5. | Unplanned admission to special (intensive) care unit | Y | N |
| 6. | Unplanned return to operating room for surgery during the same admission | Y | N |
| 7. | Ambulatory surgery patient admitted or retained for complication of surgery or anesthesia | Y | N |
| 8. | Gynecologic surgery, except radical hysterectomy or exenteration, using two or more units of blood or postoperative hematocrit of less than 24 vol% or hemoglobin of less than 8 g | Y | N |
| 9. | Unplanned removal, injury, or repair of organ during operative procedure | Y | N |
| 10. | Initiation of antibiotics more than 24 hours after surgery | Y | N |
| 11. | Discrepancy between preoperative diagnosis and postoperative tissue report | Y | N |
| 12. | Removal of uterus weighing less than 280 g for leiomyomata | Y | N |
| 13. | Removal of simple cyst or corpus luteum of ovary | Y | N |
| 14. | Hysterectomy performed on woman younger than 30 except for malignancy | Y | N |
| 15. | Gynecologic death | Y | N |

* The presence in a patient's medical record of any item on this list will be indicated by a circled "Y." This in turn will cause the patient's record to be flagged for evaluation by a physician. (Modified from a form developed by C. Irving Meeker, MD, for use at Maine Medical Center, Portland, Maine. Reprinted with permission.)

# Appendix B-3
# Sample Department Obstetric Data Summary

Provide numbers of procedures done within this hospital during the most recently completed quarter and year.

| Procedure* | Quarter<br>1 2 3 4<br>(Circle one) | Year 19 ___ |
|---|---|---|
| Patients delivered | | |
| Breech presentations, vaginal deliveries (72.5 all, except cesarean deliveries) | | |
| Forceps (72. all) | | |
| Inductions and augmentations of labor<br>    Inductions (73.4) | | |
|     Augmentations | | |
| Cesarean deliveries, total (74. all) | | |
|     Primary | | |
|     Repeat | | |
| Percentage of all births by cesarean delivery (74. all) | | |
| Attempted vaginal birth after cesarean delivery<br>    Successful | | |
|     Unsuccesful | | |

* Numbers in parentheses are ICD-9-CM codes, which may be applicable to some, but not all, procedures.

*Appendix* **B-4**
# Sample Department Gynecologic Data Summary

Provide numbers of procedures done within this hospital during the most recently completed quarter and year.

| Procedure* | Quarter<br>1  2  3  4<br>(Circle one) | Year 19 ___ |
|---|---|---|
| Gynecologic mortalities | | |
| Inpatient surgical procedures | | |
| Outpatient surgical procedures | | |
| D&Cs, not related to pregnancy (69.09)<br>    Inpatient | | |
| Ambulatory | | |
| Conizations (67.2) | | |
| Laparoscopies<br>    Sterilization (66.2) | | |
| Other (54.21) | | |
| Laser procedures<br>    Lower genital tract | | |
| Other | | |
| Hysterectomies<br>    Abdominal (68.4) | | |
| Vaginal (68.5) | | |
| Exploratory laparotomies (54.11) | | |
| Operations for urinary stress incontinence<br>    Abdominal (59.4–59.6) | | |
| Vaginal (59.3, 59.7 all) | | |

* Numbers in parentheses are ICD-9-CM codes, which may be applicable for some, but not all, procedures.

# Appendix B-5
# Sample Practitioner-Specific Obstetric Statistics

Provide numbers of procedures done within this hospital during the most recently completed quarter and year. A separate form should be completed for each physician with obstetric privileges.

Physician # _____

Specialty _____

| Procedure* | Quarter<br>1 2 3 4<br>(Circle one) | Year 19 ___ |
|---|---|---|
| Patients delivered | | |
| Breech presentations, vaginal deliveries (72.5 all, except cesarean deliveries) | | |
| Forceps (72. all) | | |
| Inductions and augmentations of labor<br>   Inductions (73.4) | | |
|    Augmentations | | |
| Cesarean deliveries, total (74. all) | | |
|    Primary | | |
|    Repeat | | |
| Percentage of all births by cesarean delivery | | |
| Attempted vaginal birth after cesarean delivery<br>   Successful | | |
|    Unsuccessful | | |

* Numbers in parentheses are ICD-9-CM codes, which may be applicable for some, but not all, procedures.

# Appendix B-6
# Sample Practitioner-Specific Gynecologic Statistics

Provide numbers of procedures done within this hospital during the most recently completed quarter and year. A separate form should be completed for each physician with privileges for any of the following procedures.

Physician # _____

Specialty _____

| Procedure* | Quarter 1 2 3 4 (Circle one) | Year 19 ___ |
|---|---|---|
| Inpatient surgical procedures | | |
| Outpatient surgical procedures | | |
| D&Cs, not related to pregnancy (69.09) Inpatient | | |
| Ambulatory | | |
| Conizations (67.2) | | |
| Laparoscopies Sterilization (66.2) | | |
| Other (54.21) | | |
| Laser procedures Lower genital tract | | |
| Other | | |
| Hysterectomies Abdominal (68.4) | | |
| Vaginal (68.5) | | |
| Exploratory laparotomies | | |
| Operations for urinary stress incontinence Abdominal (59.4–59.6) | | |
| Vaginal (59.3, 59.7 all) | | |

* Numbers in parentheses are ICD-9-CM codes, which may be applicable for some, but not all, procedures

# Appendix B-7
# Perinatal Morbidity and Mortality

Data are for 19 _____
Quarter _____

| | \multicolumn{8}{c|}{Birth weights (g)} | |
| --- | --- | --- | --- | --- | --- | --- | --- | --- |
| | 501–749 | 750–999 | 1,000–1,249 | 1,250–1,499 | 1,500–1,999 | 2,000–2,499 | >2,500 | Total for all weights |
| Number of births (all) | | | | | | | | |
| Number of perinatal deaths (fetal and neonatal deaths) | | | | | | | | |
| Fetal deaths Antepartum | | | | | | | | |
| Intrapartum | | | | | | | | |
| Neonatal deaths (<28 days) | | | | | | | | |
| Total perinatal mortality rate = Number of perinatal deaths / Number of all births | | | | | | | | _____ % |
| Neonatal autopsies performed | | | | | | | | |
| Birth trauma (all types) | | | | | | | | |

*Appendix* **B-8**
## Sample Quality Assurance Committee Activity Sheet: Individual Case Review*

Committee __QA__   Date Reviewed __8/8/88__   Chart # __123456__
Admitting Date __7/3/88__   Discharge Date __7/8/88__

1. Clinical Indicator Identified:
   1. Return to operating room for surgery--same admission
   2. Gyn surgery requiring more than 2 units of blood

2. Brief Clinical Summary:
   44-year-old, had TAH BSO for uterine myomata. Developed hemoperitoneum 3 hours postop with hypovolemic shock. Returned to operating room. Arterial bleeding noted from laceration in a small mesenteric artery secondary to retractor. Required 3 units packed cells. Did well. Discharged on 5th postop day.

3. Intensity of Injury:
   \_\_\_\_ None
   __x__ Short-term morbidity
   \_\_\_\_ Long-term morbidity
   \_\_\_\_ Mortality

4. Reviewers' Comments:
   Complication managed well when diagnosed, but complication may have been avoided if bowel examined after removal of retractor and packing.

5. Conclusions:

   \_\_\_\_ Deficiency in care — Event involving major error in diagnosis, management, judgment, or technique

   __x__ Opportunity for improvement — Event resulting from clinical situation in which management, when ideal, might have avoided the outcome

   \_\_\_\_ No deficiency identified — Management appropriate; Event due to patient's illness or unavoidable outcome

6. Committee Action:
   No trend in practitioner's performance profile noted. This incident filed in practitioner's confidential QA file for recredentialing process.

* Items 1 and 2 are completed by data abstractor; items 3–5 are completed by peer review practitioner; item 6 is completed by committee. (Designed by Robert N. Yelverton, MD, for use by the quality assurance program at Humana Women's Hospital, Tampa, Florida. Reprinted with permission.)

# Appendix B-9
# Sample Practitioner Performance Profile (Examples of Important Components)

A. Credentials

To include verification:

- Medical school: institution, location, dates, satisfactory completion
- Residency training program: institution, location, dates, specialty, satisfactory completion
- Board certification/recertification: specialty, date(s), standing (copy)
- State license(s) (copy)
- Professional liability insurance: evidence of current amount of coverage, claims settled and pending
- Current membership on other hospital staffs: evidence of standing
- Evidence of continuing medical education in field of specialty training
- Other training/experience
- Geographic proximity to hospital/prompt availability to patients
- Evidence of current health status

Written statement(s) in which the applicant agrees to:
- Abide by hospital/medical staff rules and regulations, policies, and bylaws
- Promptly report any changes in licensure, staff membership status at another hospital, felony convictions (including past convictions), health status affecting practice, final judgments or settlements in professional liability actions
- Provide for continuous care of his/her hospitalized patients

B. Clinical Privileges

- List of current privileges and dates granted/renewed
- Dates and reason for any probationary period; report on outcome/completion
- Dates and circumstances of any loss or reduction of privileges
- Any proctors' reports

C. Individual Practice Summary

Procedures: Number of key procedures performed by this physician (ie, those deemed by the department to be of particular concern; see sample forms B-3 through B-6). These numbers should be recorded on a regular basis.

Deficiencies: Number and type of deficiencies found in the cases of this physician. (These are adverse patient outcomes and deficiencies in carrying out the key procedures above as determined to be significant by peer review.) Numbers can be recorded for each key procedure the department chooses to monitor.

Percent of Deficiencies: This practitioner's deficiencies should be compared to the total number of this procedure carried out by him/her over a quarter (or year, if analysis is annual).

$$Example: \frac{\text{deficiencies in cesarean deliveries of Dr. X}}{\text{all cesarean deliveries of Dr. X}}$$

Department standing: The percentage of this practitioner's cases (by procedure or cumulative) revealing deficiencies in care compared to the department average for deficiencies (for each key procedure).

$$Example: \frac{\text{Dr. X's hysterectomy cases with deficiencies}}{\text{Department average of hysterectomy cases with deficiencies}}$$

# Appendix B-10
# *Frequency and Sources of Qualitative Data*

(This is an example of quality assurance data sources that can easily be inserted into each physician's performance profile. A chart such as this can help document how the individual practice summary was created, ie, the source of deficiencies.)

| Date / Number of deficient cases identified for this physician | Pharmacy/Therapeutics/ Drug Usage Review | Surgical Case Review | Department QA Committee | Hospital QA Committee | Infection Committee | Blood Usage Review | Medical Records Review Routine Screen/ Clinical Indicators | Procedure-Specific Criteria | Other Sources |
|---|---|---|---|---|---|---|---|---|---|
|  |  |  |  |  |  |  |  |  |  |
|  |  |  |  |  |  |  |  |  |  |
|  |  |  |  |  |  |  |  |  |  |

# Appendix C
# Uterine Size and Weight

| Type of Uterus | Size (cm) | Weight (g) |
|---|---|---|
| Normal Uterus | | |
|   Nulliparous | 5 | 70 |
|   Multiparous | 6 | 75–125 |
| Enlarged Uterus (gestational age) | | |
|   8 weeks | 6 | 125–150 |
|   12 weeks | 8 | 280–320 |
|   24 weeks | 18 | 580–620 |
|   Term | | 1,000–1,100 |

# Appendix D

# Health Care Quality Improvement Act of 1986 (42 USC §11101 et seq.)

§ 11101. Findings

The Congress finds the following:

(1) The increasing occurrence of medical malpractice and the need to improve the quality of medical care have become nationwide problems that warrant greater efforts than those that can be undertaken by any individual State.

(2) There is a national need to restrict the ability of incompetent physicians to move from State to State without disclosure or discovery of the physician's previous damaging or incompetent performance.

(3) This nationwide problem can be remedied through effective professional peer review.

(4) The threat of private money damage liability under Federal laws, including treble damage liability under Federal antitrust law, unreasonably discourages physicians from participating in effective professional peer review.

(5) There is an overriding national need to provide incentive and protection for physicians engaging in effective professional peer review.

Subchapter I—Promotion of Professional Review Activities

§ 11111. Professional review

(a) In general

(1) Limitation on damages for professional review actions

If a professional review action (as defined in section 11151(9) of this title) of a professional review body meets all the standards specified in section 11112(a) of this title, except as provided in subsection (b) of this section—

(A) the professional review body,

(B) any person acting as a member or staff to the body,

(C) any person under a contract or other formal agreement with the body, and

(D) any person who participates with or assists the body with respect to the action, shall not be liable in damages under any law of the United States or of any State (or political subdivision thereof) with respect to the action. The preceding sentence shall not apply to damages under any law of the United States or any State relating to the civil rights of any person or persons, including the Civil Rights Act of 1964, 42 USC 2000e, et seq. and the Civil Rights Acts, 42 USC 1981, et seq. Nothing in this paragraph shall prevent the United States or any Attorney General of a State from bringing an action, including an action under section 4C of the Clayton Act, 15 USC § 15C [15 USCA § 15c], where such an action is otherwise authorized.

(2) Protection for those providing information to professional review bodies

Notwithstanding any other provision of law, no person (whether as a witness or otherwise) providing information to a professional review body regarding the competence or professional conduct of a physician shall be held, by reason of having provided such information, to be liable in damages under any law of the United States or of any State (or political subdivision thereof) unless such information is false and the person providing it knew that such information was false.

(b) Exception

If the Secretary has reason to believe that a health care entity has failed to report information in accordance with section 11133(a) of this title, the Secretary shall conduct an investigation. If, after providing notice of noncompliance, an opportunity to correct the noncompliance, and an opportunity for a hearing, the Secretary determines that a health care entity has failed substantially to report information in accordance with section 11133(a) of this title, the Secretary shall publish the name of the entity in the Federal Register. The protections of subsection (a)(1) of this section shall not apply to an entity the name of which is published in the Federal Register under the previous sentence with respect to professional review actions of the entity commenced during the 3-year period beginning 30 days after the date of publication of the name.

(c) Treatment under State laws

(1) Professional review actions taken on or after October 14, 1989

Except as provided in paragraph (2), subsection (a) of this section shall apply to State laws in a State only for professional review actions commenced on or after October 14, 1989.

(2) Exceptions

(A) State early opt-in

Subsection (a) of this section shall apply to State laws in a State for actions commenced before October 14, 1989, if the State by legislation elects such treatment.

(B) State opt-out

Subsection (a) of this section shall not apply to State laws in a State for actions commenced on or after October 14, 1989, if the State by legislation elects such treatment.

(C) Effective date of election

An election under State law is not effective, for purposes of subparagraphs (A) and (B), for actions commenced before the effective date of the State law, which may not be earlier than the date of the enactment of that law.

§ 11112. Standards for professional review actions

(a) In general

For purposes of the protection set forth in section 11111(a) of this title, a professional review action must be taken—

(1) in the reasonable belief that the action was in the furtherance of quality health care,

(2) after a reasonable effort to obtain the facts of the matter,

(3) after adequate notice and hearing procedures are afforded to the physician involved or after such other procedures as are fair to the physician under the circumstances, and

(4) in the reasonable belief that the action was warranted by the facts known after such reasonable effort to obtain facts and after meeting the requirement of paragraph (3).

A professional review action shall be presumed to have met the preceding standards necessary for the protection set out in section 11111(a) of this title unless the presumption is rebutted by a preponderance of the evidence.

(b) Adequate notice and hearing

A health care entity is deemed to have met the adequate notice and hearing requirement of subsection (a)(3) of this section with respect to a physician if the following conditions are met (or are waived voluntarily by the physician):

(1) Notice of proposed action

The physician has been given notice stating—
- (A) (i) that a professional review action has been proposed to be taken against the physician,
  - (ii) reasons for the proposed action,
- (B) (i) that the physician has the right to request a hearing on the proposed action,
  - (ii) any time limit (of not less than 30 days) within which to request such a hearing, and
- (C) a summary of the rights in the hearing under paragraph (3).

(2) Notice of hearing

If a hearing is requested on a timely basis under paragraph (1)(B), the physician involved must be given notice stating—
- (A) the place, time, and date, of the hearing, which date shall not be less than 30 days after the date of the notice, and
- (B) a list of the witnesses (if any) expected to testify at the hearing on behalf of the professional review body.

(3) Conduct of hearing and notice

If a hearing is requested on a timely basis under paragraph (1)(B)—
- (A) subject to subparagraph (B), the hearing shall be held (as determined by the health care entity)—
  - (i) before an arbitrator mutually acceptable to the physician and the health care entity,
  - (ii) before a hearing officer who is appointed by the entity and who is not in direct economic competition with the physician involved, or

*Appendix D*

(iii) before a panel of individuals who are appointed by the entity and are not in direct economic competition with the physician involved;

(B) the right to the hearing may be forfeited if the physician fails, without good cause, to appear;

(C) in the hearing the physician involved has the right—

(i) to representation by an attorney or other person of the physician's choice,

(ii) to have a record made of the proceedings, copies of which may be obtained by the physician upon payment of any reasonable charges associated with the preparation thereof,

(iii) to call, examine, and cross-examine witnesses,

(iv) to present evidence determined to be relevant by the hearing officer regardless of its admissibility in a court of law, and

(v) to submit a written statement at the close of the hearing; and

(D) upon completion of the hearing, the physician involved has the right—

(i) to receive the written recommendation of the arbitrator, officer, or panel, including a statement of the basis for the recommendations, and

(ii) to receive a written decision of the health care entity, including a statement of the basis for the decision.

A professional review body's failure to meet the conditions described in this subsection shall not, in itself, constitute failure to meet the standards of subsection (a)(3) of this section.

(c) Adequate procedures in investigations or health emergencies

For purposes of section 11111(a) of this title, nothing in this section shall be construed as—

(1) requiring the procedures referred to in subsection (a)(3) of this section—

(A) where there is no adverse professional review action taken, or

(B) in the case of a suspension or restriction of clinical privileges, for a period of not longer than 14 days, during which an investigation is being conducted to determine the need for a professional review action; or

(2) precluding an immediate suspension or restriction of clinical privileges, subject to subsequent notice and hearing or other adequate procedures, where the failure to take such an action may result in an imminent danger to the health of any individual.

§ 11113. Payment of reasonable attorneys' fees and costs in defense of suit

In any suit brought against a defendant, to the extent that a defendant has met the standards set forth under section 11112(a) of this title and the defendant substantially prevails, the court shall, at the conclusion of the action, award to a substantially prevailing party defending against any such claim the cost of the suit attributable to such claim, including a reasonable attorney's fee, if the claim, or the claimant's conduct during the litigation of the claim, was frivolous, unreasonable, without foundation, or in bad faith. For the purposes of this section, a defendant shall not be considered to have substantially prevailed when the plaintiff obtains an award for damages or permanent injunctive or declaratory relief.

§ 11114. Guidelines of the Secretary

The Secretary may establish, after notice and opportunity for comment, such voluntary guidelines as may assist the professional review bodies in meeting the standards described in section 11112(a) of this title.

§ 11115. Construction

(a) In general

Except as specifically provided in this subchapter, nothing in this subchapter shall be construed as changing the liabilities or immunities under law.

(b) Scope of clinical privileges

Nothing in this subchapter shall be construed as requiring health care entities to provide clinical privileges to any or all classes or types of physicians or other licensed health care practitioners.

(c) Treatment of nurses and other practitioners

Nothing in this subchapter shall be construed as affecting, or modifying any provision of Federal or State law, with respect to activities of professional review bodies regarding nurses, other licensed health care practitioners, or other health professionals who are not physicians.

(d) Treatment of patient malpractice claims

Nothing in this chapter shall be construed as affecting in any manner the rights and remedies afforded patients under any provision of Federal or State law to seek redress for any harm or injury suffered as a result of negligent treatment or care by any physician, health care practitioner, or health care entity, or as limiting any defenses or immunities available to any physician, health care practitioner, or health care entity.

Subchapter II—Reporting of Information

§ 11131. Requiring reports on medical malpractice payments

(a) In general

Each entity (including an insurance company) which makes payment under a policy of insurance, self-insurance, or otherwise in settlement (or partial settlement) of, or in satisfaction of a judgment in, a medical malpractice action or claim shall report, in accordance with section 11134 of this title, information respecting the payment and circumstances thereof.

(b) Information to be reported

The information to be reported under subsection (a) of this section includes—

(1) the name of any physician or licensed health care practitioner for whose benefit the payment is made,
(2) the amount of the payment,
(3) the name (if known) of any hospital with which the physician or practitioner is affiliated or associated,
(4) a description of the acts or omissions and injuries or illnesses upon which the action or claim was based, and
(5) such other information as the Secretary determines is required for appropriate interpretation of information reported under this section.

(c) Sanctions for failure to report

Any entity that fails to report information on a payment required to be reported under this section shall be subject to a civil money penalty of not more than $10,000 for each such payment involved. Such penalty shall be imposed and collected in the same manner as civil money penalties under subsection (a) of section 1320a-7a of this title are imposed and collected under that section.

(d) Report on treatment of small payments

The Secretary shall study and report to Congress, not later than two years after November 14, 1986, on whether information respecting small payments should continue to be required to be reported under subsection (a) of this section and whether information respecting all claims made concerning a medical malpractice action should be required to be reported under such subsection.

§ 11132. Reporting of sanctions taken by boards of medical examiners

(a) In general

(1) Actions subject to reporting

Each Board of Medical Examiners—

(A) which revokes or suspends (or otherwise restricts) a physician's license or censures, reprimands, or places on probation a physician, for reasons relating to the physician's professional competence or professional conduct, or

(B) to which a physician's license is surrendered, shall report, in accordance with section 11134 of this title, the information described in paragraph (2).

(2) Information to be reported

The information to be reported under paragraph (1) is—

(A) the name of the physician involved,

(B) a description of the acts or omissions or other reasons (if known) for the revocation, suspension, or surrender of license, and

(C) such other information respecting the circumstances of the action or surrender as the Secretary deems appropriate.

(b) Failure to report

If, after notice of noncompliance and providing opportunity to correct noncompliance, the Secretary determines that a Board of Medical Examiners has failed to report information in accordance with subsection (a) of this section, the Secretary shall designate another qualified entity for the reporting of information under section 11133 of this title.

§ 11133. Reporting of certain professional review actions taken by health care entities

(a) Reporting by health care entities

(1) On physicians

Each health care entity which—

(A) takes a professional review action that adversely affects the clinical privileges of a physician for a period longer than 30 days;

(B) accepts the surrender of clinical privileges of a physician—

  (i) while the physician is under an investigation by the entity relating to possible incompetence or improper professional conduct, or

  (ii) in return for not conducting such an investigation or proceeding; or

(C) in the case of such an entity which is a professional society, takes a professional review action which adversely affects the membership of a physician in the society,

shall report to the Board of Medical Examiners, in accordance with section 11134(a) of this title, the information described in paragraph (3).

(2) Permissive reporting on other licensed health care practitioners

A health care entity may report to the Board of Medical Examiners, in accordance with section 11134(a) of this title, the information described in paragraph (3) in the case of a licensed health care practitioner who is not a physician, if the entity would be required to report such information under paragraph (1) with respect to the practitioner if the practitioner were a physician.

(3) Information to be reported

The information to be reported under this subsection is—

(A) the name of the physician or practitioner involved,

(B) a description of the acts or omissions or other reasons for the action or, if known, for the surrender, and

(C) such other information respecting the circumstances of the action or surrender as the Secretary deems appropriate.

(b) Reporting by Board of Medical Examiners

Each Board of Medical Examiners shall report, in accordance with section 11134 of this title, the information reported to it under subsection (a) of this section and known instances of a health care entity's failure to report information under subsection (a)(1) of this section.

(c) Sanctions

(1) Health care entities

A health care entity that fails substantially to meet the requirement of subsection (a)(1) of this section shall lose the protections of section 11111(a)(1) of this title if the Secretary publishes the name of the entity under section 11111(b) of this title.

(2) Board of Medical Examiners

If, after notice of noncompliance and providing an opportunity to correct noncompliance, the Secretary determines that a Board of Medical Examiners has failed to report information in accordance with subsection (b) of this section, the Secretary shall designate another qualified entity for the reporting of information under subsection (b) of this section.

(d) References to Board of Medical Examiners

Any reference in this subchapter to a Board of Medical Examiners includes, in the case of a Board in a State that fails to meet the reporting requirements of section 11132(a) of this title or subsection (b) of this section, a reference to such other qualified entity as the Secretary designates.

§ 11134. Form of reporting

(a) Timing and form

The information required to be reported under sections 11131, 11132(a), and 11133 of this title shall be reported regularly (but not less often than monthly) and in such form and manner as the Secretary prescribes. Such information shall first be required to be reported on a date (not later than one year after November 14, 1986) specified by the Secretary.

(b) To whom reported

The information required to be reported under sections 11131, 11132(a), and 11133(b) of this title shall be reported to the Secretary, or, in the Secretary's discretion, to an appropriate private or public agency which has made suitable arrangements with the Secretary with respect to receipt, storage, protection of confidentiality, and dissemination of the information under this subchapter.

(c) Reporting to State licensing boards

(1) Malpractice payments

Information required to be reported under section 11131 of this title shall also be reported to the appropriate State licensing board (or boards) in the State in which the medical malpractice claim arose.

(2) Reporting to other licensing boards

Information required to be reported under section 11133(b) of this title shall also be reported to the appropriate State licensing board in the State in which the health care entity is located if it is not otherwise reported to such board under subsection (b) of this section.

§ 11135. Duty of hospitals to obtain information

(a) In general

It is the duty of each hospital to request from the Secretary (or the agency designated under section 11134(b) of this title), on and after the date information is first required to be reported under section 11134(a) of this title—

(1) at the time a physician or licensed health care practitioner applies to be on the medical staff (courtesy or otherwise) of, or for clinical privileges at, the hospital, information reported under this subchapter concerning the physicians or practitioner, and

(2) once every 2 years information reported under this subchapter concerning any physician or such practitioner who is on the medical staff (courtesy or otherwise) of, or has been granted clinical privileges at, the hospital.

A hospital may request such information at other times.

(b) Failure to obtain information

With respect to a medical malpractice action, a hospital which does not request information respecting a physician or practitioner as required under subsection (a) of this section is presumed to have knowledge of any information reported under this subchapter to the Secretary with respect to the physician or practitioner.

(c) Reliance of information provided

Each hospital may rely upon information provided to the hospital under this chapter and shall not be held liable for such reliance in the absence of the hospital's knowledge that the information provided was false.

§ 11136. Disclosure and correction of information

With respect to the information reported to the Secretary (or the agency designated under section 11134(b) of this title) under this subchapter respecting a physician or other licensed health care practitioner, the Secretary shall, by regulation, provide for—

(1) disclosure of the information, upon request, to the physician or practitioner, and

(2) procedures in the case of disputed accuracy of the information.

§ 11137. Miscellaneous provisions

(a) Providing licensing boards and other health care entities with access to information

The Secretary (or the agency designated under section 11134(b) of this title) shall, upon request, provide information reported under this subchapter with respect to a physician or other licensed health care practitioner to State licensing boards, to hospitals, and to other health care entities (including health maintenance organizations) that have entered (or may be entering) into an employment or affiliation relationship with the physician or practitioner or to which the physician or practitioner has applied for clinical privileges or appointment to the medical staff.

(b) Confidentiality of information

(1) In general

Information reported under this subchapter is considered confidential and shall not be disclosed (other than to the physician or practitioner involved) except with respect to professional review activity, as necessary to carry out subsections (b) and (c) of section 11135 of this title (as specified in regulations by the Secretary), or in accordance with regulations of the Secretary promulgated pursuant to subsection (a) of this section. Nothing in this subsection shall prevent the disclosure of such information by a party which is otherwise authorized, under applicable State law, to make such disclosure. Information reported under this part that is in a form that does not permit the identification of any particular health care entity, physician, other health care practitioner, or patient shall not be considered confidential. The Secretary (or the agency designated under section 11134(b) of this title), on application by any person, shall prepare such information in such a form and shall disclose such information in such form.

(2) Penalty for violations

Any person who violates paragraph (1) shall be subject to a civil money penalty of not more than $10,000 for each such violation involved. Such penalty shall be imposed and collected in the same manner as civil money penalties under subsection (a) of section 1320a-7a of this title are imposed and collected under that section.

(3) Use of information

Subject to paragraph (1), information provided under section 11135 of this title and subsection (a) of this section is intended to be used solely with respect to activities in the furtherance of the quality of health care.

*Appendix D*

(4) Fees

The Secretary may establish or approve reasonable fees for the disclosure of information under this section or section 11136 of this title. The amount of such a fee may not exceed the costs of processing the requests for disclosure and of providing such information. Such fees shall be available to the Secretary (or, in the Secretary's discretion, to the agency designated under section 11134(b) of this title) to cover such costs.

(c) Relief from liability for reporting

No person or entity (including the agency designated under section 11134(b) of this title) shall be held liable in any civil action with respect to any report made under this subchapter (including information provided under subsection (a) of this section) without knowledge of the falsity of the information contained in the report.

(d) Interpretation of information

In interpreting information reported under this subchapter, a payment in settlement of a medical malpractice action or claim shall not be construed as creating a presumption that medical malpractice has occurred.

Subchapter III—Definitions and Reports

§ 11151. Definitions

In this title:

(1) The term "adversely affecting" includes reducing, restricting, suspending, revoking, denying, or failing to renew clinical privileges or membership in a health care entity.

(2) The term "Board of Medical Examiners" includes a body comparable to such a Board (as determined by the State) with responsibility for the licensing of physicians and also includes a subdivision of such a Board or body.

(3) The term "clinical privileges" includes privileges, membership on the medical staff, and the other circumstances pertaining to the furnishing of medical care under which a physician or other licensed health care practitioner is permitted to furnish such care by a health care entity.

(4) (A) The term "health care entity" means—

　　(i) a hospital that is licensed to provide health care services by the State in which it is located,

　　(ii) an entity (including a health maintenance organization or group medical practice) that provides health care services and that follows a formal peer review process for the purpose of furthering quality health care (as determined under regulations of the Secretary), and

　　(iii) subject to subparagraph (B), a professional society (or committee thereof) of physicians or other licensed health care practitioners that follows a formal peer review process for the purpose of furthering quality health care (as determined under regulations of the Secretary).

(B) The term "health care entity" does not include a professional society (or committee thereof) if, within the previous 5 years, the society has been found by the Federal Trade Commission or any court to have engaged in any anti-competitive practice which had the effect of restricting the practice of licensed health care practitioners.

(5) The term "hospital" means an entity described in paragraphs (1) and (7) of section 1395x(e) of this title.

(6) The terms "licensed health care practitioner" and "practitioner" mean, with respect to a State, an individual (other than a physician) who is licensed or otherwise authorized by the State to provide health care services.

(7) The term "medical malpractice action or claim" means a written claim or demand for payment based on a health care provider's furnishing (or failure to furnish) health care services, and includes the filing of a cause of action, based on the law of tort, brought in any court of any State or the United States seeking monetary damages.

(8) The term "physician" means a doctor of medicine or osteopathy or a doctor of dental surgery or medical dentistry legally authorized to practice medicine and surgery or dentistry by a State (or any individual who, without authority holds himself or herself out to be so authorized).

(9) The term "professional review action" means an action or recommendation of a professional review body which is taken or made in the conduct of professional review activity, which is based on the competence or professional conduct of an individual physician (which conduct affects or could affect adversely the health or welfare of a patient or patient), and which affects (or may affect) adversely the clinical privileges, or membership in a professional society, of the physician. Such term includes a formal decision of a professional review body not to take an action or make a recommendation described in the previous sentence and also includes professional review activities relating to a professional review action. In this chapter, an action is not considered to be based on the competence or professional conduct of a physician if the action is primarily based on—

(A) the physician's association, or lack of association, with a professional society or association,

(B) the physician's fees or the physician's advertising or engaging in other competitive acts intended to solicit or retain business,

(C) the physician's participation in prepaid group health plans, salaried employment, or any other manner of delivering health services whether on a fee-for-service or other basis,

(D) a physician's association with, supervision of, delegation of authority to, support for, training of, or participation in a private group practice with, a member or members of a particular class of health care practitioner or professional, or

(E) any other matter that does not relate to the competence or professional conduct of a physician.

(10) The term "professional review activity" means an activity of a health care entity with respect to an individual physician—

(A) to determine whether the physician may have clinical privileges with respect to, or membership in, the entity,

(B) to determine the scope or conditions of such privileges or membership, or

(C) to change or modify such privileges or membership.

(11) The term "professional review body" means a health care entity and the governing body or any committee of a health care entity which conducts professional review activity, and includes any committee of the medical staff of such an entity when assisting the governing body in a professional review activity.

(12) The term "Secretary" means the Secretary of Health and Human Services.

(13) the term "State" means the 50 States, the District of Columbia, Puerto Rico, the Virgin Islands, Guam, American Samoa, and the Northern Mariana Islands.

(14) the term "State licensing board" means, with respect to a physician or health care provider in a State, the agency of the State which is primarily responsible for the licensing of the physician or provider to furnish health care services.

§ 11152. Reports and memoranda of understanding

(a) Annual reports to Congress

The Secretary shall report to Congress, annually during the three years after November 14, 1986, on the implementation of this chapter.

(b) Memoranda of understanding

The Secretary of Health and Human Services shall seek to enter into memoranda of understanding with the Secretary of Defense and the Administrator of Veterans' Affairs to apply the provisions of subchapter II of this chapter to hospitals and other facilities and health care providers under the jurisdiction of the Secretary or Administrator, respectively. The Secretary shall report to Congress, not later than two years after November 14, 1986, on any such memoranda and on the cooperation among such officials in establishing such memoranda.

(c) Memorandum of understanding with drug enforcement administration

The Secretary of Health and Human Services shall seek to enter into a memorandum of understanding with the Administrator of Drug Enforcement relating to providing for the reporting by the Administrator to the Secretary of information respecting physicians and other practitioners whose registration to dispense controlled substances has been suspended or revoked under section 824 of Title 21. The Secretary shall report to Congress, not later than two years after November 14, 1986, on any such memorandum and on the cooperation between the Secretary and the Administrator in establishing such a memorandum.

# Appendix E
# Quality Assurance in ACOG

Quality assurance efforts within the American College of Obstetricians and Gynecologists (ACOG) are multidimensional. The primary thrust rests with two task forces, each composed of seven physicians and one nurse. One task force oversees ACOG's peer review program, Voluntary Review of Quality of Care (VRQC), and the other addresses broad aspects of quality assurance within this medical specialty.

In the Voluntary Review of Quality of Care Program, specially trained Fellows of ACOG and nurse members of NAACOG serve as peer reviewers for hospital departments of obstetrics and gynecology that request a department-wide evaluation. Review teams summarize their findings in a comprehensive report and make recommendations based on their analysis of hospital data and patient records, tour of the facility, and interviews with key hospital staff. The overseeing national level task force establishes guidelines and methodology, trains reviewers, and examines reports submitted by the hospital review teams. The program operates on a fee-for-service basis. Participating hospitals are billed for College administrative costs and reviewers' services.

Members of the Task Force on Quality Assurance were appointed by ACOG's Executive Board with the charge of determining and addressing the needs of the Fellowship within the area of quality assurance. The task force, which commenced planning for this manual in late 1986, drafted the original clinical indicators, monitoring systems, and criteria sets included in this manual. The narrative text was also written by members of the Task Force on Quality Assurance. The manual is intended to replace ACOG's 1981 publication *Quality Assurance in Obstetrics and Gynecology*.

# Appendix F
# Bibliography

American Academy of Pediatrics, American College of Obstetricians and Gynecologists. Guidelines for perinatal care. 2nd ed. Washington, DC: AAP, ACOG, 1988

American College of Obstetricians and Gynecologists. Standards for obstetric-gynecologic services. 7th ed. Washington, DC: ACOG, 1988

American Hospital Association. Verification of physician credentials. Technical Advisory Bulletin. Chicago, Illinois: AHA, 1985

American Hospital Association. Privileges and quality assurance for nonphysician practitioners. AHA Policy and Statement. Chicago, Illinois: AHA, 1987

American Hospital Association. Quality assurance management in a hospital. AHA Guidelines. Chicago, Illinois: AHA, 1983

American Hospital Association. Utilization review in health care institutions. AHA Policy and Statement. Chicago, Illinois: AHA, 1981

American Medical Association. A compendium of state peer review immunity laws. Chicago, Illinois: AMA, 1988

American Medical Association. Bylaws: a guide for hospital medical staff. Chicago, Illinois: AMA, 1984

American Medical Association, Council on Medical Service. Quality of care. JAMA 1986;256(8):1032–1034

Bernstein AH. Hospital medical staff: privileges and procedures. Hospitals 1981;55(7):62, 65–66

Donabedian A. Criteria and standards for quality assessment and monitoring. QRB, 1986;12(3):99–108

Eisele CW, Fifer WR, Wilson TC. The medical staff and the modern hospital. Englewood, Colorado: Estes Park Institute, 1985

Fineberg KS. Obstetrics/Gynecology and the law. Ann Arbor, Michigan: Health Administration Press, 1984

Geiersbach SA. Revocation of staff privileges: due process responsibilities. Mich Hosp 1983;19(3):13–16

Inglehart JK. Congress moves to bolster peer review: the health care quality improvement act of 1986. N Engl J Med 1987; 316(15):960–964

Joint Commission on Accreditation of Healthcare Organizations. Accreditation manual for hospitals, 1989. Chicago, Illinois: JCAHO, 1988

Joint Commission on Accreditation of Healthcare Organizations. Examples of monitoring and evaluation in obstetrics and gynecology. Chicago, Illinois: JCAHO, 1988

Joint Commission on Accreditation of Healthcare Organizations: Medical staff, monitoring and evaluation: departmental review. Chicago, Illinois: JCAHO, 1988

Joint Commission on Accreditation of Hospitals (Healthcare Organizations). Risk management and quality assurance: issues and interactions. QRB. Chicago, Illinois: JCAHO, 1986

Joint Task Force on Hospital-Medical Staff Relationships. The report of the Joint Task Force on Hospital-Medical Staff Relationships. American Hospital Association, American Medical Association. Chicago, Illinois, 1985

Lang DA, Hopkins JL. Trustees' responsibility for professional standards. QRC Advisor 1988;4(7):4–6

Meisenheimer CG, ed. Quality assurance: a complete guide to effective programs. Rockville, Maryland: Aspen, 1985

Singer AR, Schnier SV. Initiating the corrective action process. QRC Advisor 1987;3(4):1–7

U.S. Congress Office of Technology Assessment. The quality of medical care: information for consumers, OTA-H-386. Washington, DC: US Government Printing Office, 1988

# Appendix G
# Other ACOG Publications

In its continuing effort to ensure a high quality of practice and to educate Fellows and their patients, the American College of Obstetricians and Gynecologists (ACOG) has developed a variety of educational materials. These include practice guidelines, professional development programs, and patient information materials. A description of some of these publications or resources follows:

- *Standards for Obstetric–Gynecologic Services, seventh edition.* The first edition of *Standards* was published in 1959. This publication sets forth recommendations and suggests guidelines for the provision of obstetric and gynecologic health care services in a variety of institutions by a variety of practitioners. The purpose of *Standards* is to provide guidelines that will ensure a basic level of care as well as a continuum of obstetric–gynecologic care, no matter where within the health care system or by whom care is provided. They are presented as recommendations and general guidelines rather than as a body of rigid rules and are intended to be adapted to many different situations, according to the needs and resources particular to the locality, the institution, or type of practice. Variations and innovations that demonstrably improve the quality of patient care are to be encouraged rather than restricted. *Standards* do not, by and large, discuss the management of clinical conditions.

- *Guidelines for Perinatal Care, second edition.* A supplement to the ACOG *Standards*, this publication emphasizes a regional approach to perinatal care. Jointly published by ACOG and the American Academy of Pediatrics, it suggests practice guidelines for obstetric and neonatal care.

- *Technical Bulletins.* Information bulletins are designed to provide practicing obstetricians and gynecologists with new information on practice, procedures, and clinical management of diseases. They are educational in nature and are not intended to constitute standards.

- *ACOG Committee Opinions.* Opinions prepared by ACOG practice committees usually address clinical issues of emerging or specialized interest.

- *ACOG Statements of Policy.* Executive board-approved statements of policy provide official policy on particular topics, including clinical care issues.

- *Precis III: An Update in Obstetrics and Gynecology.* This publication summarizes in a single volume current information about the specialty and its clinical application, with emphasis on recent advances.

- *PROLOG: Personal Review of Learning in Obstetrics and Gynecology.* This self-assessment program series focuses on diagnostic and management problems in obstetrics, gynecology, reproductive endocrinology and infertility, clinical gynecologic oncology, and patient management in the office.

- *Patient Education Pamphlets and Booklets.* Designed to answer patients' questions on current procedures and issues in obstetrics and gynecology, this series is particularly beneficial in keeping patients informed of and involved in their health care.

Publications can be ordered by calling ACOG's Resource Center at (202) 863-2518 and requesting an order form. Order forms may be sent to:

ACOG Distribution Center
PO Box 91180
Washington, DC 20090-1180
Telephone: (703) 683-1774

# Glossary of Terms

*Abstract:* To glean from a medical record particular items of clinical data about a patient and the medical care that she received.

*Agenda for Change:* Initiated in 1986, a program of the Joint Commission on the Accreditation of Healthcare Organizations, which emphasizes the assessment of actual patient *outcomes* rather than the *capacity* of each health care facility to deliver good quality of care.

*Accreditation:* The official certification of an institution, by an external organization, that the institution meets a certain standard or specific requirements. A hospital must be accredited before it can receive Medicare reimbursement or offer resident training. The Joint Commission on the Accreditation of Healthcare Organizations is the primary accrediting agency for health care organizations.

*Antepartum:* Prior to the onset of labor.

*Appropriateness:* The degree of correlation between a condition and the action taken to improve it. In order to be appropriate, medical care should be provided in the proper time frame, amount, duration, and level of intensity. It should also be acceptable to the presumably well-informed person receiving it.

*Audit:* A qualitative review (or comparison) of patients' medical charts focusing on a single physician's care or a single procedure or diagnosis. Qualitative findings are classified and tabulated relative to the focus and time frame of the audit.

*Clinical Indicator:* A measurable dimension (eg, a medical event, procedure, diagnosis, or outcome) that is thought to reflect an important aspect of medical care. Clinical indicators are used as part of a screening process (ie, a simple review of medical records for a few specific facts) to make some preliminary determinations about the quality of care.

*Comorbidity:* The existence of two or more clinical conditions simultaneously, increasing the patient's need for medical services.

*Complication:* An untoward patient event, occurrence, or outcome that results from or follows treatment.

*Concurrent Audit/Review:* An evaluation of medical care that takes place while care is still being provided (ie, prior to patient discharge) as opposed to after the fact. The presumed superiority of a concurrent audit over a retrospective audit is that intervention can occur. Utilization of services is often the target of concurrent review.

*Credentialing:* The process of reviewing the qualifications, education, and previous relevant experiences of an individual applying for appointment or reappointment to practice medicine in an institution. Delineation of clinical privileges (see privilege delineation) is part of this process.

*Criteria/Criteria Sets:* Something that should or should not occur in relation to a medical event (ie, a standard against which clinical activity can be compared for the purpose of evaluation). ACOG criteria are designed as minimum standards of acceptable care.

*Death:* For the purpose of quantifying hospital mortalities, any death occurring within 6 weeks of a diagnostic or therapeutic procedure.

*Deficiency:* A variation in practice that represents inadequate judgment, skill, or performance; deviation from accepted norms or care that does not meet preset criteria (eg, a primary cesarean delivery done for failure to progress without labor).

*Diagnosis-Specific:* Something that is related to a particular diagnosis rather than to any diagnosis (eg, lack of variability is specific to the diagnosis of fetal distress).

*Discovery:* Pretrial procedures to inform the participants of evidence in order to minimize the element of surprise at the time of trial. These typically include interrogatories and depositions, but can also include requests for admission of facts and requests for genuineness of documents.

*Due Process:* Those particular steps that allow an individual to challenge what he or she views as an inappropriate, adverse decision. Each hospital's bylaws should clearly delineate the system of due process for that institution. Written, timely notification by the hospital of allegations, as well as an objective hearing process, are two steps required under due process.

*Duty:* An obligation recognized by the law. A health care professional's duty to a patient is to provide the degree of care ordinarily exercised by health care professionals who practice in the same clinical specialty and under similar circumstances.

*Exception:* A deviation from the normal decision/treatment process that is judged to be acceptable. Exceptions should be clearly documented in medical records, and the reason for an approach different from the norm or accepted treatment should be explained.

*Expert Opinion:* The testimony of a person who has special training, knowledge, skill, or experience in an area relevant to the resolution of a legal dispute.

*Febrile Morbidity:* An oral temperature of 38.0°C (100.4°F) on at least 2 postoperative days, excluding the first 24 hours after surgery.

*Fetal Distress:* A compromise in fetal physiology. Although the term "fetal distress" is included in this manual because it is often used and therefore familiar, it is not a sufficiently accurate description of fetal condition.

*Focused (problem-oriented) Audit/Review:* The evaluation of a specific aspect of medical care (eg, all abdominal hysterectomies performed over the course of 1 year) to determine whether there is a deficiency and, if so, what its nature and cause are, and what corrective methods are most likely to resolve it. The initial problem may be identified by any of a variety of quality assurance triggers in place to detect variations in care. Continued monitoring to determine the effectiveness of any action taken is recommended.

*Generic Screen:* General elements of medical care and patient outcomes that can be easily extracted from medical records for the purpose of identifying those cases that may require peer review to determine whether medical care was deficient. These are neither diagnosis-specific nor procedure-specific. The clinical indicators included in this manual are, in most cases, generic screens.

*ICD-9-CM (International Classification of Diseases, Ninth Revision, Clinical Modifications):* Lists and corresponding codes for diseases and procedures. This was the source of the code numbers assigned to procedures and indications within criteria sets provided in this manual.

*Incident Report:* The official written report of an untoward event that occurred in an institution. Usually the event is directly related to patient care and interaction with the staff. If there is a continuing problem or risk, prompt documentation, and correction must be undertaken by the institution.

*Indication:* The reason for carrying out a particular process or procedure.

*Indicator:* A measurable dimension of an important aspect of clinical care; an event, action, occurrence, or outcome (eg, a laboratory result) associated with a particular clinical event (see *clinical indicator*).

*Informed Consent:* A legal process that requires a physician to obtain the patient's consent for treatment rendered or an operation performed. Without an informed consent, the physician may be held liable for violation of the patient's rights, even if the treatment was appropriate and rendered with due care.

*Intrapartum Death:* The death of a fetus during labor.

*Justification:* A clinically valid reason for a failure to follow preset criteria; the determination, often through peer review, that care was acceptable although some aspect of patient care was different from that outlined in preestablished criteria.

*Life-Threatening Event:* Any intraoperative or postoperative cardiac or respiratory arrest, cerebrovascular accident, myocardial infarction, pulmonary embolus, shock, or coagulopathy.

*Locality Rule:* The traditional rule requiring that an expert witness practice in the same community as the defendant. This rule has now been superceded in most states by a national standard of care.

*Maloccurrence:* An untoward clinical event.

*Malpractice:* Professional negligence. In medical terms, malpractice is the failure to exercise the degree of care that is used by reasonably careful health care professionals of like qualifications in the same or similar circumstances. The failure to meet this acceptable standard of care is malpractice only if it causes the patient injury.

*Monitor (n):* A tool with which to evaluate clinical care (similar to an indicator); an incremental bit of clinical data that is examined because of the information that it is expected to convey about broader practice patterns and quality.

*Monitor (v):* To track the occurrence of specified, important events and analyze trends that emerge over time. Monitoring is undertaken as part of the process of creating practitioner and department performance profiles.

*National Standard of Care:* The degree of care and skill expected of a reasonably competent practitioner in the same specialty acting under similar circumstances.

*Negligence:* A legal cause of action arising from the failure to exercise the degree of diligence and care that a reasonable and ordinarily prudent person would exercise under the same or similar circumstances.

*Neonatal Mortality:* The death of a liveborn infant up to 28 days after birth (up to and including 27 days, 23 hours, and 59 minutes from the moment of birth).

*Outcome:* An end point. Outcome evaluation focuses on the patient's health status after actions have been taken and treatment has been provided.

*Outcome Audit:* A study of a patient's medical records to assess the effect of treatment provided on the patient's health.

*Outliers:* Variations from the norm. In quality assurance programs, outliers are cases that do not fit the established criteria and thus require further investigation before the quality of care can be determined.

*Pattern of Care:* An overview of the medical care provided to patients by a practitioner. This overview often involves compiling quantifiable patient data and comparing them to patient data from other practitioners.

*Peer Review:* An evaluation or review of the performance of colleagues by professionals with similar types and degrees of expertise (eg, the evaluation of one physician's practice by another physician). True peer review must be conducted by a professional with the same type of training as the professional being reviewed.

*Peer Review Organizations (PRO):* A type of organization created by federal legislation in 1984 (as the successor to professional standards review organizations, or PSRO) to review the utilization, appropriateness, and quality of hospital care. A primary responsibility is to determine the appropriateness of care to Medicare beneficiaries. Payment can be denied if care provided is deemed inappropriate.

*Perinatal Mortality:* The death of a fetus or live-born infant who survived only briefly (not more than 28 days). Although perinatal mortality is often reported according to age, weight-specific reporting that categorizes weights into 500-g increments is encouraged because it is more accurate than are age-specific reporting categories.

*Practitioner Performance Profile:* Also referred to as physician profile or practice profile. A comprehensive record of the clinical events, procedures, and outcomes that occurred over time in a single provider's practice. The purpose of profiling is to discern patterns or trends in volume, quality, and appropriateness of care in the individual's practice. A practitioner's performance profile can be compared or combined with those of others to form an overview or profile of the entire department. When statistical information on practice patterns and quality assurance findings are combined with other important data unique to each physician (such as credentials), a complete picture of the physician emerges.

*Privilege Delineation/Privileging:* The act of granting an individual the right to perform specific diagnostic or therapeutic procedures within an institution. Each practitioner's level and type of privileges must be specified. The basis for hospital approval of a practitioner's request for privileges must be the applicant's education, training, experience, and demonstrated ability in each relevant area.

*Postpartum:* Immediately following delivery.

*Process:* The way in which something is done; the mechanisms and resources brought to bear on a problem or task.

*Process Audit:* An evaluation of clinical activities and resources to determine whether appropriate steps were taken in patient care. Process audits are often contrasted with outcome audits, which focus on the impact of activities and resources on patients' health status.

*Glossary of Terms*

*Proctoring:* Immediate oversight during a clinical procedure, especially a surgical procedure, of a practitioner by a physician viewed as an expert in the procedure being performed. Proctors are expected to report, usually to the department head, on the quality of performance that they observe. Granting of privileges, delineation of specific privileges, or satisfactory completion of a provisional or probationary period may be contingent upon a favorable written report from a proctor. In some instances, proctoring may take the form of medical record review rather than direct observation.

*Professional Liability:* The legal responsibility of a health care provider to his or her patient. Health care providers are presumed to owe a duty to the patients under their professional care and may be liable to charges of medical malpractice if injury results from their failure to perform with the same degree of skill and knowledge that any competent practitioner with similar training would exhibit in a similar situation.

*Prospective Audit/Review:* A review occurring at the time of (or immediately following) the delivery of medical services. Such a review often takes the form of utilization review or preadmission screening to determine the status of a patient and the appropriateness of the proposed use of resources and level of medical care. Third-party providers often use this method to review admissions and thus control access/costs.

*Quality:* The essence of something's nature or degree of excellence. In order to determine the level of quality in an attempt to ensure "high quality," it is necessary first to determine the criteria or standards against which comparisons can be made.

*Quality Assurance System:* A system and process to provide ongoing monitoring and evaluation of the health care offered by an institution and its providers.

*Readmission:* Any unplanned rehospitalization within 6 weeks (42 days) of surgery because of a complaint or problem related to the primary operation.

*Retrospective Audit/Review:* An evaluation of medical care after its provision, usually after the patient has been discharged.

*Review:* A formal evaluation of medical care provided. Reviews may be prospective, concurrent, or retrospective. At the preliminary screening level, reviews may be conducted by nonphysicians according to predetermined clinical indicators. When a patient record is flagged by the screening process, the final determination of quality is made by physician peers. A review is similar to, but broader than, an audit.

*Risk Management:* The steps taken, usually following an untoward event, to decrease the possibility of a malpractice action being initiated and to prevent ensuing loss (see *incident report*).

*Risk Prevention:* Actions taken to decrease the chance that an untoward event will occur (ie, ensuring that care is of the highest quality possible). This includes the identification and reduction or elimination of threats and risks.

*Screen:* A tool used for review (eg, a clinical indicator).

*Screening:* The process of reviewing charts for some predetermined, presumably important and representative, aspect of care. Assumptions about the quality or patterns of care are often based on findings from screening a sample of medical records.

*Standard of Care:* Norms of behavior and action as defined by a particular profession (eg, nurse practice acts, policies, procedures, guidelines). Standards may reflect optimal or threshold levels of care, rather than what the majority views as appropriate. The criteria sets in this manual are threshold levels, rather than normative or optimal levels.

*Threshold Level:* The base or minimum acceptable level; often perceived as a starting point. Criteria in this manual are intended to represent care below which most physicians would agree that care is unacceptable.

*Transfusion:* Any intraoperative or postoperative administration of whole blood or blood products.

*Trends:* Ongoing or repetitive patterns of care.

*Trending:* The process of comparing data collected over a period of time so that quality can be judged on the basis of a number of significant events.

*Unplanned Surgery:* Any surgical procedure for correcting a complication directly related to surgery. Corrective surgery may be performed either interoperatively or postoperatively during the same hospitalization.

***Untoward Event:*** Any occurrence that is undesirable and usually unexpected, such as an adverse patient outcome.

***Utilization Review:*** An evaluation and determination of the appropriateness of a patient's use of medical care resources. Reviews may occur at any point in the health care system (eg, prospective approval prior to entry, concurrent review during an inpatient stay, or retrospective review after services were provided).

***Variation:*** Something that is different from the expected or mandated process or outcome. Variations in practice reflect differences from previously established criteria for patient care.